T0196350

# Endorsements

*Whether you are the person who is stuck and can't get well, or the person who is well but never wants to get sick, I wholeheartedly recommend this stellar education as a hidden cause of chronic disease that is not only preventable but correctable.*

**-Sherry A. Rogers**, M.D., ABEM, ABFP, FACAAI, FACN, Clinician and Author of *Detoxify Or Die, How To Cure Diabetes, Is Your Cardiologist Killing You?*, and more.

*"Poisoned? What You Don't Know About Heavy Metals Is Killing You," by Dr. Pamela Owens is a breakthrough encapsulation of a modern day epidemic. What we showed in the $31 million National Institute of Health, double blind, randomized, 132 center chelation trial, TACT (trial to assess chelation therapy) extremely positive results and safety I believe was directly a result of the detoxification effects of heavy metals, especially lead. Reads easily, even for the general public. I highly recommend it!*

**-Roy Heilbron,** M.D., Cardiologist, Author, TACT Trial Researcher, see YouTube: https://www.youtube.com/watch?v=6UyDmDdfEjU

*This is one of the most- timely and informative books I've ever read. I commend Dr. Owens for her investigative research. Her sincerity and passion for empowering the public is evident throughout. Toxic heavy metals surround us every single day and it's important to understand where they're coming from and what you can do about it to prevent chronic disease and disastrous health problems. This book is a MUST READ!*

*- **Dr. Matthew Loop**, Author, Speaker, Social Media Revenue Strategist*

*As I was quoted in Dr. Pamela Owens' Poisoned! What You Don't Know About Heavy Metals is Killing You, there is a predictable way that the body breaks down and a methodical way you can test and correct all these issues. This work outlines what everyone needs to know about the ways that our body breaks down when it is exposed to heavy metals, and the methodical way that we can help correct this heavy metal burden. Through sharing her journey of health and hardships that many are bound to identify with, Dr. Owens' provides a thorough account of the sources, mechanisms, and symptoms of heavy metal exposure. Her step-by-step program to overcoming heavy metal exposure lends itself to a manual that everyone can read, yet is backed by scientific facts and reputable sources- a hard feat to accomplish. It is a highly important piece of literature in emphasizing the omnipresent but little known threat of heavy metals that we are all faced with and the importance of keeping up with general health in order to combat these harsh toxins.*

**-Dr. Daniel Kalish, Founder of: The Kalish Method, Author and Researcher**

# POISONED!

## What You Don't Know About Heavy Metals Is Killing You!

### Environmental Toxic Heavy Metals:
### The Hidden Reason You Feel Sick

## Dr. Pamela J Owens

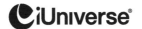

**Poisoned! What You Don't Know About Heavy Metals Is Killing You!**
**Environmental Toxic Heavy Metals: The Hidden Reason You Feel Sick**

*iUniverse books may be ordered through booksellers or by contacting:*

*iUniverse*
*1663 Liberty Drive*
*Bloomington, IN 47403*
*www.iuniverse.com*
*1-800-Authors (1-800-288-4677)*

*ISBN: 978-1-4917-8795-3 (sc)*
*ISBN: 978-1-4917-8796-0 (e)*

*Library of Congress Control Number: 2016902356*

*Print information available on the last page.*

*iUniverse rev. date: 03/28/2016*

"Unless you know what you are fighting,
how can you expect to formulate
a strategy to defeat it?"

-Dr. Pat Sullivan (Author of *Wellness Piece by Piece*)

# Table of Contents

# List of Tables

# Foreword by Dr. Ron Grisanti

Dr. Pamela J. Owens' newest book, *Poisoned! What You Don't Know About Heavy Metals Is Killing You!* is a must read for all.

The health consequences from heavy metal toxicity are occurring at epidemic rates.

The main threats to human health from heavy metals are associated with exposure to lead, cadmium, mercury and arsenic and other less common metals. These metals have been extensively studied and their effects on human health thoroughly reviewed by international bodies such as the World Health Organization (WHO).

Unknown to many, the effects of multiple heavy metal exposure, or synergistic effects are rarely evaluated by primary physicians. Scientists and researchers have joined forces and are letting the medical community know that heavy metals have serious and far-reaching consequences.

Pervasive heavy metals have been found to disrupt the immune, nervous, and endocrine systems. As more people are exposed to these toxicants there continues to be increases in infertility, certain cancers, developmental delays, asthma, chemical sensitivities, and hormonal imbalances. Heavy metals have been implicated in causing and exacerbating many of these conditions.

Every day millions of people are unknowingly exposed to heavy metals and unfortunately our bodies cannot metabolize and clear all of them. Chemicals not metabolized are stored in the fat cells throughout our bodies, where they continue to accumulate. As these chemicals build up they alter our metabolism, cause enzyme dysfunction and nutritional deficiencies, create hormonal imbalances, damage brain chemistry and can cause cancer.

As mentioned above, heavy metals are dangerous because they tend to **bioaccumulate**. Bioaccumulation means an increase in the concentration of a chemical in a biological organism over time, compared to the chemical's concentration in the environment. Because the chemicals accumulate in different parts of the body—at different rates and in different combinations—there are many different chronic illnesses that can result.

The presence of heavy metals can be a burden, hindering patients from responding to treatment. Practitioners searching for a patient's underlying causes of illness should consider testing for these toxicants as a priority in their assessment.

Although "heavy metal" toxicities due to lead, mercury, and cadmium are generally considered rare in mainstream medicine, heavy metal literate healthcare providers disagree and recognize that chronic accumulation may in fact contribute to adverse health effects.

Dr. Owens' new book is a detailed blueprint helping the patient and forward thinking healthcare professionals identify the specific heavy metal toxic burden and determine an effective and optimal treatment to decrease the toxic load.

Dr. Owens has compiled an outstanding manuscript for both the lay person interested in learning more about heavy metal toxicity and the healthcare professional desiring a road map in the diagnosis and treatment of heavy metals.

# CHAPTER 1

# Introduction-Why you need this book!

## My Story

The health problems that result from toxic heavy metal exposure affect all of us—and yes, I mean you! None of us are exempt from the slow, but cumulative deteriorating changes in health that result from being exposed to heavy metals year after year. Many of us are told that our health problems are the result of normal disease processes, or maybe they just come with age, or genetics—the list of possible misdiagnoses goes on and on. The unfortunate truth is that the effects of heavy metal poisoning are all too often misdiagnosed. Heavy metals mimic just about every common disease that sends you to the doctor's office. It is a scary fact that heavy metals don't discriminate. They just do what they do--year after year, until your health is compromised. Most doctors never even question you as to where you grew up, or where you worked, nor do they ask about possible environmental exposures. Questions such as whether or not you drank well water, or whether you were exposed to leaded gasoline or paints are seldom asked. So, consequently, you have never been tested for toxic heavy metal exposure. The good news is that finally the trend is changing. Those of us who practice Functional Health Medicine are doing our best to educate and get the "word out." Having an understanding of this tremendous health issue will hopefully stimulate your personal concern and drive you to be tested. Once your baseline heavy metal toxicity is established by checking the bioaccumulation of heavy metals and toxic load, we can set up a treatment plan, work to clean it out of your body thru detoxification, teach you to clean up your personal environment and limit your future exposure. This leads to a much healthier and happier life!

My personal story may be a lot like yours. I never thought in a million years that a toxic heavy metal load was causing some of my health issues. Who … me? After all, I called myself the "health queen"! Wow, did I have a lot to learn! My journey has been remarkable and life changing. I am happy that I can share with you some of the facts I have learned and hope it encourages you and those you love to ***get tested for heavy metals!***

As a child growing up on a farm in the South I sure had a lot of fun! I have many memories of riding on the tractor and combine with my father as he sprayed pesticides for the bugs that ate our crops. We grew many crops including tobacco, which was routinely sprayed with arsenic (Yes, arsenic!). Back then, there were no warnings about the toxicity of these chemicals. We used our hands and sticks to stir--no gloves, no protection. We syphoned gasoline (yes, with our mouths!) from the pick-up truck to put in the lawn mowers and go-carts. We drank well water that was leaching from the dirty downstream river and the pipes into the house were cast iron and lead. Back then, we just simply "had no clue" of how bad all this really was for our health.

Needless to say, the lead from the pipes ended up in my bones. In addition, I often suffered from stomach issues and avoided a lot of food because of it. I was tagged a "picky eater" and was hyperactive in school. Years later, after seeing several dermatologists, I was diagnosed with eczema when I continually broke out in rashes year after year. Prescriptions never helped so I just lived with the discomfort and pain. Many years ago, while in practice, I stumbled upon an article about gluten intolerance and I realized that I had all of the listed symptoms. What I did not know at the time was that the gluten, along with the toxic heavy metal load I had no idea I was carrying, had basically destroyed my ability to absorb vitamins and minerals. I had leaky gut and malabsorption issues. So, I proceeded to have special tests done and realized that gluten had been causing my eczema all along. I cleaned up my diet by removing—and the rash went away! What's more, I no longer suffered from bloating, lost weight, and overall felt the best I had felt in years! (Please check out great books written on this subject by: JJ Virgin, Dr. William Davis, Dr. David Perlmutter and Dr. Peter Osborne (also known as the "Gluten Warrior")). I told everyone about this latest discovery and urged testing for celiac disease, gluten intolerance and sensitivities! This was the beginning of my journey into Alternative Medicine treatments. Today it has expanded into Functional Health Medicine, a field of medicine in which I am proud to be a part. Practitioners of functional medicine focus on the real "root cause" of what is actually causing the symptoms of a condition. We don't drug you up and mask the symptoms.

Perhaps like many of you, I have moved several times since childhood. I have traveled to different states and stayed under different living conditions (apartments, condos, old moldy houses/ basements, and new homes). At times I have lived in the country, at times in the city. Heavy metal exposure has affected my life through copper pipes, toxic well water, air pollution from the local steel mill, textile manufacturers puffing soot into the air and water, and fishing in the trout streams with local toxic waste runoff. This is in addition to the many tick,

> "I was living on a nutritionally sound diet with all the best supplements. I cringe to think how bad it might have been had I been living on the standard American diet!"

spider, and mosquito bites causing their own set of problems, including biotoxins and inflammation; not to mention complications from "sick building" and mold issues along the way. Over the years, these invisible hazards creep up on you and interrupt the delicate pathways your body uses to keep you healthy.

Several years ago, I began suffering with muscle and joint pain, which wasn't too surprising considering the long hours I stand during work. However, following these symptoms came the fatigue, brain fog, insomnia and vertigo. Every doctor I saw said, "you are getting older," or "it's your hormones, you know you are getting closer to menopause." I thought holy cow-if this is how I am feeling in my forties, my fifties are going to be a nightmare! At this time, I had access to top herbal and alternative treatments, all of which gave periodic symptom relief but in time, many returned. I had test after test performed by various physicians. Intuitively, I knew there was something more to my symptoms. When all the tests came back normal, I was forced to resign myself to living with the discomfort. It is important to mention that I was living on a nutritionally sound diet with all the best supplements! I cringe to think how bad it might have been had I been living on the "standard American diet"!

Once while traveling out of town, I began experiencing moderate neck and back pain and contacted a local Chiropractor for treatment. As fate would have it, I saw Dr. Ron Grisanti. He is the founder of Functional Medicine University, and also practices Functional Medicine. As we discussed my symptoms, he recommended a heavy metals test. Meanwhile, I researched everything on this issue and agreed that this was most likely at least part of my puzzling health problems.

My test results were shocking! My lead levels were 8 times normal, aluminum was 4 times normal, mercury was 5 times normal and copper was 3 times normal! When I realized that most of my health symptoms were directly related to heavy metal toxicity, I was relieved to know that there was a "real reason" for them.

I knew immediately that I needed to "detoxify" the heavy metals from my body. I started oral chelation therapy the first year and I retested every 6 months. As the levels decreased, I cut back on the chelation dose. It has taken time, but over the years, the levels have dropped significantly (remember these levels are cumulative and are affected by where we have lived and our environmental exposure--so the load is different for each of us). I also had to detoxify my personal environment. Pots and pans, aluminum cans, cosmetics, toiletries, glassware, flat ware—sources for exposure surround us.

I continue to retest every 8-10 months since I cannot completely control the environment and the problem is not going away--we are exposed to more toxicants every year. Regular testing gives me a "heads up" in case I have been exposed to another contaminant so I can get it chelated before it has a chance to cause big problems.

There is so much wonderful information available from doctors I respect, such as: Dr. Garry Gordon, Dr. Sherry Rogers, Dr. Mark Hyman, Dr. Roy Heilbron, Dr. Norman Shealy, Dr. Joe Mercola, Dr. Richard Horowitz, Dr. Datis Kharrazian and many others. Currently, I have teamed up with Dr. Daniel Kalish of "The Kalish Method" to learn even more about toxic heavy metals and how they are the "stealers of health."

Toxic heavy metal contamination is "**one piece**" to the environmental puzzle. For some, it is an enormous piece, for others--a smaller piece. We must remember that inflammation, chronic fatigue, muscle and joint pains, depression, insomnia, neuralgias, and many other symptoms are caused by environmental issues that have merely been overlooked over the years. Health issues can start from other sources not considered, such as moldy/water and damaged "sick buildings" and homes that people have worked and lived in for years breathing in toxic spores. Lyme disease also causes symptoms that mimic those of heavy metal toxicity. A simple tick bite from an infected tick may be carrying infectious agents such as: *Babesia, Bartonella* or *Ehrlichia.* Most of the standard lab testing that is done is not sensitive enough to detect these infections. These infections, along with the overlap of other issues one may have been exposed to, set off chronic illnesses and create **M**ultiple **S**ystemic **I**nfectious **D**isease **S**yndrome (**MSIDS**) as discovered by Dr. Richard Horowitz and written about in his latest book "Why Can't I Get Better?" Therefore, it is imperative to seek advice from those who know the correct tests to run. Not to mention, there are more and more new bugs being discovered that coat cells with biofilm and damage them by releasing biotoxins. These can take years to diagnose, and usually after going to many, many Doctors, and having numerous testing procedures done, as well as having spent hundreds of dollars, some may finally get the right diagnosis and treatment.

Many of the above conditions require specialized tests, which should be performed by trained experts in the field. If you are interested in being tested, outside of myself, I recommend Dr. Sonia Rapaport, Chapel Hill, NC and Dr. Richard Horowitz Hyde Park, NY to name a couple. There are more Doctor's listed in the Resource section at the end of the book.

Therefore, being an expert on toxic heavy metals, and having firsthand knowledge on this issue, I present the book: "Poisoned! What You Don't Know About Heavy Metals Is Killing You! How to Overcome The Hidden Reason You Feel Sick." This book is to be used as an educational guide, for you to gain knowledge, and to help empower your decision making in order to conquer this invisible problem. Please get tested and tell those you love to do the same! I look forward to helping you along your journey to decrease the heavy metal toxicity many of us have encountered, by no fault of our own.

## Who Will Benefit from this Book?

Heavy metal poisoning does not discriminate. Heavy metals are toxic to virtually all forms of life and are found throughout the environment. What's more, potential exposures are increasingly more common in this industrial age. Needless to say, this book is for everyone. Anyone living on this planet runs the risk of heavy metal poisoning, making the information provided in the following pages vital for identify potential sources and reducing or eliminating potential exposures. Advice about what to do if you have already been exposed is also included. The chapters in this book are logically arranged to provide you with information about the most dangerous heavy metals and where you are most likely to be exposed to them. Then, a simple plan for alleviating the symptoms associated with current and past exposures is given, along with strategies for avoiding future problems. Also included are real abstracts from cutting-edge research currently being done as well as other research-related tidbits.

## The Problem Explained

Many heavy metals are toxic. Plus, they can be found lurking everywhere in our environment. Heavy metals are used in a wide range of applications from fertilizers to cosmetics to pharmaceuticals. It is also becoming increasingly difficult to avoid exposure to many toxic heavy metals as they are incorporated into our industrial society at alarming rates.

But, how common is it to suffer from heavy metal poisoning? If we take a look at history, it is easy to see that exposure to heavy metals is not a new concept. It is possible that the fall of the Roman Empire was at least in some part affected by the presence of high levels of lead in the drinking water. Similarly, the term "mad as a hatter" was coined from workers in the hat industry who developed neurological problems because mercury was a main ingredient in the manufacturing process.

**Today, heavy metals have corrupted our food supply, our water, some pharmaceuticals, cosmetics, imported food products, herbs and supplements, and in many cases even the air we breathe.**

The question, then, is not whether or not you have been exposed to heavy metals, but rather which ones and how much? It is now known that even trace amounts of some heavy metals can result in adverse health effects, some of which may be misdiagnosed as mental conditions such as aggressive and anti-social behavior. One of the many ways in which heavy metals can wreak havoc on your body include such insidious mechanisms as being an "anti-nutrient" in which the heavy metals actually deplete your body of other vital nutrients. Others metals "mimic" the activity of essential minerals-- causing important pathways for proper health to become confused and disrupted. Still other heavy metals contribute to oxidative stress, providing a constant supply of "free radicals" that actively work to age and destroy your system.

It is a fact that we can inherit the toxic burden of our parents. Scientists call these inheritable changes to our DNA "epigenetics," and they can affect every aspect of our health—*and* be passed down to our children and then grandchildren. Mothers can also directly pass toxicants to their offspring while still in the womb and later through breast milk. Sadly, when blood taken from the umbilical cords of newborn infants was analyzed for common environmental toxicants, 287 different compounds were detected. The authors of this study said this:

> *"... of the 287 chemicals we detected in umbilical cord blood, we know that 180 cause cancer in humans or animals, 217 are toxic to the brain and nervous system, and 208 cause birth defects or abnormal development in animal tests"* **(Environmental Working Group 2005)**

To compound the issue, after birth you are continually adding new exposures through interactions with your environment according to where you live (or have lived), worked, whether you drink well water or city water (each have their own issues), your proximity to hazardous industry practices that spew contamination into the air and/or water and consumption of contaminated foods from all over the world--grown in cultures without environmental standards in place. The list is endless. Now, years of exposure to toxic heavy metals have accumulated to the point that your body is no longer able to adequately manage them and you are experiencing various symptoms and health problems. Perhaps you have tried medical procedures or medication after medication (stents, bypass surgeries, antidepressants or other antipsychotics, etc.) but you are still suffering from symptoms such as a lack of sex drive, fatigue, insomnia, vertigo, muscle and joint pain, osteoporosis, peripheral neuropathies, weight gain, diabetes, memory loss, brain fog and the list goes on. Perhaps the doctors have implied it is all in your head! Or, you are told to chalk it up to genetics or simply aging. Sound familiar?

**But, no one has ever tested you for heavy metals! These dangerous toxicants are invisible to us and this is why we must "get out of the box" and get tested for these "stealers of health"!**

In this book, we will discuss the most dangerous heavy metals as well as where they come from, why they are dangerous, and how they adversely impact your health. Then, we will explore our natural detoxification system and why it is being overwhelmed by the sheer quantity of toxicants that it is required to deal with on a daily basis. Finally, we will discuss ways you can counteract exposure to heavy metals and support your body's natural detoxification system, **test your toxic load for baseline markers and most of all, prevent heavy metals from adversely affecting your health in the future.**

> "Air pollution and water pollution are only part of the story. There are thousands of harmful environmental toxins, some of which we are aware of, such as pesticides, chemicals, household cleaners–and others, which seem perfectly innocent, such as those ubiquitous plastic water bottles, styrene cups, dental fillings and plastic wrap. These are just a few small examples of the alarming amount of harmful toxins our bodies are absorbing every day."
>
> -Dr. Sherry Rogers
> (Clinician, Researcher, and Author of several books including: *Detoxify Or Die*.)

# Chapter 1 References

Environmental Working Group, 2005. "Body burden: the pollution in newborns." Environmental Working Group Accessed September 30, 2014. http://www.ewg.org/research/body-burden-pollution-newborns.

# CHAPTER 2

# Mercury

Mercury is perhaps one of the best known and most feared of all the toxic heavy metals. It certainly deserves this reputation. The presence of mercury in our food supply is one of the most disturbing cases of a toxic heavy metal that is infiltrating our lives. You only have to monitor the behavior of the US Food and Drug Administration (FDA) in regards to mercury in order to understand that its presence in the environment has become a significant problem. In fact, the FDA maintains an ongoing list of foods that should not be consumed *at all* by high-risk populations and only in moderation by everyone else. Unfortunately, the issues with mercury do not just stop with our supply of seafood and even freshwater fish. Now, mercury is finding its way into other ecosystems and wreaking equally devastating havoc.

Even at sub-lethal doses, mercury is causing overwhelming losses to species other than just aquatic animals. It has long been known that fish eating birds are vulnerable to high levels of mercury, but researchers are now discovering that songbirds consuming insects from polluted water sources are suffering severe health issues as well. The affected bird populations are undergoing reduced reproductive success, hormonal changes, suppressed immune systems and loss of location-based memory (needed to find food sources) (Langley 2014). That sounds a lot like the common medical complaints of millions of Americans! In addition, other animals relying on insects for food are similarly affected. Bats for example have been found to contain levels of mercury so high that it resulted in behavioral changes (Mercola 2014a). In humans, the list of health problems associated with mercury exposure is only getting longer. Unfortunately, many people respond so differently to mercury exposure that it can be very difficult to diagnose without adequate testing.

## Common Sources of Mercury Exposure

One of the most widely known sources for mercury exposure is through the consumption of fish. Fish accumulate mercury in the tissues of their body when they are exposed to it in aquatic environments that become contaminated, primarily from coal-burning power plants (Mozaffarian 2009). The burning of coal releases mercury into the air, which can then be deposited into water sources through acid rain. There are other industrial practices that may contribute to increases in environmental mercury levels as well, such as cement kilns and certain mining activities. To make matters worse, bacteria that are found in the water can convert the mercury that is released from industrial sources into a form that is especially dangerous to biological organisms—called methylmercury. It is methylmercury that accumulates in fish. Large predatory fish tend to accumulate the most methylmercury because their primary source of food is mercury-contaminated smaller fish. It is important to remember, however, that even small levels of mercury can disrupt the sensitive systems of your body that help to maintain good health. That is why consumption of any type of fish should be done with caution and only through verified, reputable vendors of mercury-free fish (see table 1 for mercury levels in commonly consumed seafood). For a free online calculator to estimate how much mercury you are consuming, visit http://seaturtles.org/programs/mercury/.

**Common Sources for Mercury**

Inorganic:
- Dental Amalgams
- Fish
- Coal-burning plants
- Cement Kilns
- Chlor-alkali plants (manufacture bleach, laundry detergent, PVC, etc.)
- Some sources of high fructose corn syrup
- Gold mining
- Fluorescent (energy efficient) light bulbs

Organic:
- Fish (methylmercury)
- Vaccines (primarily flu)
- Polluted waterways

*Dr. Pamela J Owens*

Table 1. Mercury levels in commonly consumed seafood.

| Fish | Median Mercury (ppm) |
| --- | --- |
| Tilefish | 1.450 |
| Swordfish | 0.995 |
| Shark | 0.979 |
| Mackerel | 0.730 |
| Tuna | 0.689 |
| Orange Roughy | 0.571 |
| Marlin | 0.485 |
| Grouper | 0.448 |
| Bluefish | 0.368 |
| Sablefish | 0.361 |
| Albacore Tuna | 0.358 |
| Halibut | 0.241 |
| Weakfish | 0.235 |
| Monkfish | 0.181 |
| Snapper | 0.166 |
| Bass | 0.152 |
| Perch | 0.150 |
| Cod | 0.111 |
| Carp | 0.110 |
| American Lobster | 0.107 |

A second source of mercury exposure that is not as widely known is through the dental practice of using mercury as a medium for filling cavities, known as mercury dental amalgams. In fact, mercury dental amalgams are the number one source for mercury exposure in the United States (Mercola 2011)! This is made especially alarming because of the close proximity of the mercury fillings to the brain. It is important to understand that under the conditions that exist in your mouth, mercury will continually release "vapors" that can easily pass through a membrane called the "blood brain barrier." The blood brain barrier is the body's most important defense against environmental influences because it is especially difficult for typical compounds—including many drugs—to pass through. In fact, a single mercury dental amalgam can release as much as 6 times the amount of mercury that is found in contaminated seafood. **With such easy access to the brain, it is no wonder why so many Americans are experiencing adverse health effects from mercury fillings.**

It has been well documented that the mercury found in routine dental amalgams release a constant amount of mercury into your mouth, which can then travel to other areas of your body. This is why the removal of mercury dental amalgams is critical for people who are suffering from mercury toxicity. However, if done improperly, having mercury amalgams removed can actually cause a significant amount of harm. Fortunately, there are a number of dentists throughout the country who have been specially trained in the removal of mercury dental amalgams safely. Key questions you can ask your dentist about their methods for removing the mercury from your mouth in order to ensure that your dentist is adequately trained include the following (Adapted from (McGuire 2005)):

- What are your methods for keeping the mercury cool while you are drilling? *The heat caused by drilling increases the release of mercury, both as a vapor and as mercury particles. Most dentists who have been properly trained in the removal of mercury amalgams use a process called "chunking," which involves less drilling and the use of special tools to remove the mercury in chunks.*
- Do you use a high-volume evacuator?
  *An important tool for minimized the risk associated with the removal of mercury amalgams is a high-volume evacuator that has a more powerful suction system than what is used by most dentists.*
- Do you use an additional air-filtration system?
  *An additional air-filtration system placed as close to the patient's mouth as possible may reduce exposure to the outgassing of mercury vapors that may occur during removal.*
- Will you provide me with an alternative source of air during the procedure?
  *This is important for minimizing the amount of mercury vapors you are inhaling during the procedure. Your dentist should instruct you to breathe through your nose and avoid "mouth-breathing" during the procedure.*

- Will you use a rubber dam during the procedure?
  *A rubber dam will isolate the tooth or teeth that are being worked on and helps to minimize accidental exposure during the procedure.*

You can find more information on how to find a dentist who has been trained in the safe removal of mercury amalgams in the resource section at the end of the book.

## Mercury and Cardiovascular Disease

"This [Mercury] in fact may be the missing piece of the puzzle in reducing high blood pressure." Research has shown that exposure to mercury can increase the risk of developing cardiovascular disease, including high blood pressure (hypertension) and atherosclerosis (coronary artery disease) (Mozaffarian 2009)(Salonen et al. 1995). Unfortunately, information about the role that mercury plays in the development of cardiovascular disease is complicated by information on the positive effects of consuming fish for improving heart health. Since we know that the primary source of dietary mercury comes from fish, the question remains should we consume fish or not?

> "This [Mercury] in fact may be the missing piece of the puzzle in reducing high blood pressure."
>
> -Dr. Ronald Grisanti (Author and President of Functional Medicine University)

According to a recent geological survey, 100 percent of the fish tested in fresh water environments were contaminated with mercury (Scudder et al. 2009). This means that it is not just large, salt-water fish that pose a risk—but, virtually all fish. What's more, when the incidence of cardiovascular disease was measured in men who were commonly exposed, even small levels of mercury were related to an increase in hypertension (Skoczynska et al. 2010). While the consumption of omega-3 fatty acids found in fish is definitely beneficial, consuming even small amounts of mercury may counteract the positive effects (Salonen et al. 1995). So, consumption of wild fish caught in remote areas that have been verified free of mercury contamination is the best option if you want to continue eating fish. Otherwise, taking a high quality fish oil supplement is a good alternative for supplying the necessary omega-3 fatty acids for improving heart health without the negative effects of mercury.

## Mercury and Prenatal Risks

There are few things as important to parents as the health of their child(ren). That's why the risk posed by mercury to an unborn child is especially worrisome. Early development in the womb is a critical time for the nervous system and all other organs to develop correctly. It can also set the stage for how their small bodies will interact with and handle the many challenges they will face in the environment once they are born. It is a big responsibility. Unfortunately, we know that when an unborn child is exposed to mercury the risk of neurological or development disorders is greatly increased. Neurological damage that occurs in the womb can result in delayed walking and talking, as well as a shortened attention span or even a learning disability (Suzuki et al. 2010). **This can happen when the mother consumes contaminated food such as fish, through mercury dental amalgams, handling a broken thermometer, contact with and breathing fumes from broken mercury-containing light bulbs and many other sources.** Mothers who have a high number of mercury dental amalgams, in particular, may put their unborn child at risk for developmental problems such as autism (Geier, Kern, and Geier 2009). If the mother is exposed to high enough levels of mercury, it can cause severe birth defects and possibly result in the baby being stillborn (Missouri Department of Natural Resources, 2014). Once the baby is born, it is still important to monitor exposure to mercury—especially if the mother is breastfeeding. It has been shown that mercury can be passed to the infant not only through the umbilical cord and directly through the placenta, but also in breast milk once the baby is born (Yang et al. 1997). Other common practices, such as chewing gum, can also increase the release of mercury from

15

dental amalgams—potentially increasing the exposure to the unborn or nursing child.

## Mercury and the Nervous System

The nervous system is more sensitive to mercury exposure than any other organ system in the body. Clearly, exposure to mercury in very young people can lead to devastating neurological problems that will continue throughout life. It is important to realize that adult exposure to mercury is not without consequences. People who are regularly exposed to mercury in the workplace, for example, commonly complain of chronic fatigue, volatile emotions, tremors, and a tendency for increased inflammation (Tang and Li 2006). Mercury cannot enter the brain through the circulatory system because it is unable to cross the blood brain barrier; however, studies in fish have demonstrated that mercury can instead travel directly to the brain through the nerves themselves (Mercola, 2014b). The presence of mercury in the central nervous system leads to devastating consequences through psychological, neurological and even immunological pathologies that contribute to a long list of health problems. Combine this with the fact that by age two, American children have exceeded the EPA's designated "safe" level for mercury exposure 2,000 fold! Unfortunately, the problem is compounded by the extremely long half-life (15–30 years) of mercury in the central nervous system unless it is actively removed (Mercola, 2014b). Other health problems that may be indirectly related to mercury's effects on the nervous system include: kidney damage, autoimmune conditions, cognitive decline, mouth ulcers and periodontal diseases. These are all symptoms that can cause a dramatic decrease in the quality of life, yet are very difficult for doctors to determine the cause without appropriate heavy metal testing; therefore, appropriate treatment is rare or sometimes harmful. For example, a recent case study highlighted the lack of awareness for mercury poisoning when a woman was misdiagnosed with multiple sclerosis that was in fact mercury poisoning. She only started to recover after conducting her own research and insisting she be tested for heavy metals (Parry 2014).

## Mercury and Autism

The causes of autism tend to be highly contentious among people in differing medical fields. There is emerging evidence about the role of mercury, however, that is difficult to ignore. Correlations have been made between the number of mercury dental amalgams in mothers and the risk—and even severity—of autistic symptoms in their children (Geier, Kern, and Geier 2009). It is not a simple issue. Exposure to mercury also causes changes in gene expression in autistic boys that do not occur in boys who show typical development. This means that children with certain genetics have a higher risk for developing autism if they are exposed to mercury than children who have slightly different genes (Geier, Kern, and Geier 2009). This might also explain why there is so much confusing literature on the safety of vaccines—what is relatively harmless for one child might result in mild to serious autistic characteristics in another child. At this point, the safest option for parents is to avoid exposing their child(ren) to any type of mercury. This might include vaccines that are known to contain mercury as well as fish. Mercury containing dental amalgams should be avoided at all costs! Also, regular check-ups to monitor mercury levels and actively treating any exposure are important for prevention of any long-term disorders.

## Mechanisms of Mercury Toxicity

Researchers are continually discovering new information about the ways in which mercury causes disease in humans. Some of the best-known pathways include:

- By causing the formation of free radicals and oxidative stress
- By Inhibiting the body's natural defenses against oxidative stress
- By causing damage to lipids that are circulating in the blood, which can contribute to cardiovascular disease
- By disrupting the body's normal blood clotting functions, especially dangerous for those with a high risk of stroke or with other blood abnormalities

- By changing the architecture of the nervous system—resulting in developmental and neurological damage
- By inducing mitochondrial dysfunction, which impairs the body's ability to produce energy from food

## Key Points about Mercury

- Consumption of wild fish caught in remote areas that have been verified free of mercury contamination is the best option if you want to continue eating fish.
- Taking a high quality fish oil supplement is a good alternative for supplying the necessary omega-3 fatty acids for improving heart health without the negative effects of mercury.
- Parents should avoid exposing their child(ren) to any type of mercury. This might include vaccines that are known to contain mercury as well as fish.
- Mercury containing dental amalgams should be avoided at all costs.

## Chapter 2 References

Missouri Department of Natural Resources. 2014. "Mercury can affect human health." Accessed September 17, 2014. http://www.dnr.mo.gov/env/mercury-impact.htm.

Geier, D. A., J. K. Kern, and M. R. Geier. 2009. "A prospective study of prenatal mercury exposure from maternal dental amalgams and autism severity." *Acta neurobiologiae experimentalis* 69 (2):189-97.

Langley, C. 2014. "W&M biologists find link between mercury dosage, songbird losses." http://www.vagazette.com/news/va-vg-mercury-in-birds-051714-20140516,0,6325775.story.

McGuire, T. 2005. "How to remove mercury amalgam (silver) dental fillings." Accessed December 22, 2014. http://www.mercuryfreenow.com/freeservices/amalremov.html.

Mercola, J. 2011. "Still carrying around mercury next to your brain?" Accessed September 19, 2014. http://articles.mercola.com/sites/articles/archive/2011/09/04/mercury-poisoning-from-silver-fillings.aspx.

Mercola, J. 2014a. "Environmental mercury tied to increasing songbird losses." Accessed September 15, 2014. http://articles.mercola.com/sites/articles/archive/2014/06/10/songbird-mercury-pollution.aspx.

Mercola, J. 2014b "Mercury toxicity and systemic elimination agents." Accessed September 27, 2014. http://www.mercola.com/article/mercury/mercury_elimination.htm.

Mozaffarian, D. 2009. "Fish, mercury, selenium and cardiovascular risk: current evidence and unanswered questions." *International journal of environmental research and public health* 6 (6):1894-916. doi: 10.3390/ijerph6061894.

Parry, L. 2014. "Woman with 'toxic dental fillings' discovers mercury poisoning is to blame for crippling symptoms mistaken for MS." Accessed September 27, 2014. http://www.dailymail.co.uk/health/article-2703896/Woman-toxic-dental-fillings-discovers-mercury-poisoning-blame-crippling-symptoms-mistaken-MS.html.

Salonen, J. T., K. Seppanen, K. Nyyssonen, H. Korpela, J. Kauhanen, M. Kantola, J. Tuomilehto, H. Esterbauer, F. Tatzber, and R. Salonen. 1995. "Intake of mercury from fish, lipid peroxidation, and the risk of myocardial infarction and coronary, cardiovascular, and any death in eastern Finnish men." *Circulation* 91 (3):645-55.

Scudder, B.C., L.C. Chasar, D.A. Wentz, N.J. Bauch, M.E. Brigham, P.W. Moran, and D.P. Krabbenhoft. 2009. Mercury in fish, bed sediment, and water from streams across the Unites States, 1998-2005. edited by U.S. Department of the Interior.

Skoczynska, A., M. Jedrejko, H. Martynowicz, R. Poreba, A. Affelska-Jercha, A. Steinmetz-Beck, B. Turczyn, A. Wojakowska, and I. Jedrychowska. 2010. "[The cardiovascular risk in chemical factory workers exposed to mercury vapor]." *Medycyna pracy* 61 (4):381-91.

Suzuki, K., K. Nakai, T. Sugawara, T. Nakamura, T. Ohba, M. Shimada, T. Hosokawa, K. Okamura, T. Sakai, N. Kurokawa, K. Murata, C. Satoh, and H. Satoh. 2010. "Neurobehavioral effects of prenatal exposure to methylmercury and PCBs, and seafood intake: neonatal behavioral assessment scale results of Tohoku study of child development." *Environmental research* 110 (7):699-704. doi: 10.1016/j.envres.2010.07.001.

Tang, N., and Y. M. Li. 2006. "Neurotoxic effects in workers of the clinical thermometer manufacture plant." *International journal of occupational medicine and environmental health* 19 (3):198-202.

Yang, J., Z. Jiang, Y. Wang, I. A. Qureshi, and X. D. Wu. 1997. "Maternal-fetal transfer of metallic mercury via the placenta and milk." *Annals of clinical and laboratory science* 27 (2):135-41.

# CHAPTER 3

# Aluminum

Aluminum is probably best known for its place in the soda pop industry or as a common item found in many kitchens throughout the United States--from the all-purpose "tin-foil" to aluminum pans. That's why it might come as a surprise to many people that aluminum is actually a very dangerous heavy metal that is contributing to the overall decline in health that is pervasive in our society. Aluminum is a very common component of the earth's crust, and often makes its way into the air, soil and water systems. Consider, however, that our bodies have absolutely no use for aluminum and even though it is a "natural" substance, it is also a potently toxic heavy metal. In recent years, aluminum has replaced mercury as an adjuvant in many childhood vaccines. Adjuvants are used alongside the vaccine itself in order to stimulate the immune response and, hopefully, enhance its effectiveness. As a potent neurotoxicant, aluminum exposure is definitely worth avoiding, especially as it is capable of traveling to the brain and forming "deposits" that are extremely difficult to remove. Also, aluminum may interfere

## Common Sources for Aluminum

- Aluminum cans
- Cookware (baking/ cooking pans, foil, etc.)
- Food additives (processed cheese, table salt, baking powders, pickles, bleached flour, prepared dough, cake mixes, non-dairy creamers, vanilla powders and some donuts and waffles, baby formulas)
- Cigarette filters
- Vaccines
- Some medications (such as antacids and nasal sprays)
- Pesticides
- Personal care items (such as antiperspirant)

with the body's ability to cope with any type of mercury exposure—making aluminum and mercury partners in crime!

## Common Sources for Aluminum Exposure

Aluminum may be one of the most difficult of all heavy metals to avoid. It is found everywhere in the environment and easily makes its way to our food and water supplies and can also be found in the air and soil. To compound the problem, it is a common agent in the manufacturing of many common items such as "pop cans," cooking pans, aluminum foil and as an additive in many foods and even medical supplies—including infant formulas, baking soda, vaccines, and parenteral preparations.

## The Aluminum Alzheimer's Connection

Nobody wants to get sick. But, on the continuum of feared and dreaded diseases, Alzheimer's tops the list—superseded only by cancer. Many people have experienced or witnessed the devastation that Alzheimer's disease can bring to a family and even whole communities. Yet, the outlook is not as hopeless as people are led to believe. Scientists are making important discoveries about the causes of Alzheimer's every day, one of the most important of which is the role of aluminum; and steps can be taken to avoid and treat exposures!

Ironically, the role of aluminum in the development of Alzheimer's disease has been heavily disputed at times—despite its reputation as the most abundant heavy metal on earth that is known to have neurotoxic properties. It is also hard to ignore the fact that aluminum can act as a neurotoxicant at very low levels, and in fact most people consume enough aluminum in their diet to meet the limit needed for aluminum toxicity. Not only that, but **scientists have repeatedly shown that persons who have been positively diagnosed with Alzheimer's disease have an unusually high level of aluminum that has accumulated in their neurons!** Studies dating back as early as 1911 have shown that long-term exposure to aluminum will cause the hallmark symptoms of Alzheimer's disease (Tomljenovic 2011). The circumstantial evidence supporting a role for aluminum in Alzheimer's disease has been accumulating for years. Interestingly, a recent case study from northeast England demonstrated that an individual exposed to high levels of aluminum that later died of Alzheimer's disease also had high levels of aluminum in the brain. Authors claim that this is the first case that directly demonstrates a link between aluminum and Alzheimer's disease (Medical News Today, 2014). It is not necessary to sit around with a "wait and see" attitude about whether or not you will get Alzheimer's disease. Exposure to aluminum can be avoided. Previous exposures can be treated, but action is required!

## Aluminum and Autism

Research has shown a very tight association between autism spectrum disorders and aluminum-containing vaccines (Shaw and Tomljenovic 2013). So, why do U.S. health officials still insist that American kids be so heavily vaccinated? There are various reasons for this: 1) vaccine advocates argue that aluminum is poorly absorbed by the body and therefore poses a low risk of toxicity 2) vaccine advocates argue that the amount of aluminum given through vaccines is generally less than what a typical child will be exposed to through everyday consumption of contaminated food and water, and 3) vaccine advocates argue that the public health benefits of childhood vaccinations outweigh the risks to any one individual. But, how accurate are these arguments? First, all arguments have to be placed within the proper context. While it may be true that aluminum consumed via food and water is poorly absorbed, the same does **NOT** apply to aluminum that is given through a parenteral injection such as the typical vaccine shot. This route of exposure bypasses many of the obstacles presented by the gut that may slow down the absorption of aluminum systemically into the body. Also, it is well known that the infant gut does not function the same way as a mature adult. The gastrointestinal tract of infants, are "leaky" by design in order for the baby to absorb the antibodies given in the mother's milk to assist with those first encounters with pathogens. So, while a healthy adult may not absorb a significant amount of aluminum through the gut—the same may not be true of infants. Similarly, it is dangerous to assume that levels of aluminum that appear to be safe in food and water are equally safe when injected directly into the body (for the same reasons discussed above), especially given the accumulative properties of aluminum in the body. Finally, the rates of autism and autism spectrum disorders are skyrocketing in this country. If, indeed, there is a correlation between aluminum-containing vaccines and the high rates of autism, then the true question becomes exactly how does the public benefit? Researchers from the Neural Dynamics Research Group in Canada expressed the concern like this:

> Experimental research, however, clearly shows that aluminum adjuvants have a potential to induce serious immunological disorders in humans. In particular, aluminum in adjuvant form carries a risk for autoimmunity, long-term brain inflammation and associated neurological complications and may thus have profound and widespread adverse health consequences (Tomljenovic and Shaw 2011).

## Aluminum and the Skeletal System

It is frightening to consider that common household items such as aluminum and lead can actually replace calcium in bone—resulting in abnormal mineralization patterns that can lead to a long list of health problems. The intestines can absorb aluminum after it has been consumed and it is then rapidly carried in the blood to bone repositories and dumped. Once aluminum makes it way to the bone, it can be stored for long periods of time and therefore has a tendency to accumulate (Malluche 2002). For this reason, even short-term exposure to aluminum may contribute to long-term diseases as the aluminum slowly builds up in the body. Therefore, ingestion of aluminum should be avoided whenever possible.

So what does it mean when aluminum accumulates in the bones? Calcium is essential for maintaining the density and strength of bones. So, it is no surprise that bone strength is dramatically decreased when a significant amount of calcium has been replaced with aluminum and the risk of suffering from a fragility fracture increases at the same time. Interestingly, persons with Alzheimer's disease also have an unusually high number of bone fractures—most likely due to excessive aluminum that has deposited in their bones over a lifetime (Mjoberg et al. 1997).

## Aluminum and Kidney Disease

Aluminum is excreted from the body primarily via the kidneys in the urinary output. For this reason, patients with any kind of kidney (renal) insufficiency are at an increased risk for developing other symptoms due to aluminum toxicity. The impaired elimination of aluminum through the kidneys leads to accumulation in other body organs such as the brain and bone. As we mentioned earlier, increased aluminum in the nervous system will lead to documented symptoms that are very similar to those observed in Alzheimer's patients. In fact, the term "dialysis dementia" has been coined to describe dialysis patients that suffer from aluminum toxicity (Wills and Savory 1989).

## Mechanisms of Aluminum Toxicity

Researchers are continually discovering new information about the ways in which aluminum causes disease in humans. Some of the best-known pathways include:

- Aluminum is a known neurotoxin that poses a significant risk for long-term damage to the nervous system
- Aluminum is able to "fool" the body into replacing calcium in the bones—resulting in a weak skeletal system
- Aluminum very likely causes an abnormal immune response and may contribute to autoimmune diseases
- Aluminum interferes with the normal uptake and distribution of iron in the blood. Iron is a necessary component of hemoglobin, the protein which carries oxygen from the lungs to the rest of the body

## Key Points about Aluminum

- Even short-term exposure to aluminum may contribute to long-term diseases as the aluminum slowly builds up in the body. Therefore, ingestion of aluminum should be avoided whenever possible.
- The circumstantial evidence supporting a role for aluminum in Alzheimer's disease has been accumulating for years.
- Patients with any kind of kidney (renal) insufficiency are at an increased risk for developing other symptoms due to aluminum toxicity.

## Chapter 3 References

Medical News Today. 2014. "Elevated brain aluminum and early onset Alzheimer's disease in an individual occupationally exposed to aluminum." Accessed September 19, 2014. http://www.medicalnewstoday.com/releases/272573.php.

Malluche, H. H. 2002. "Aluminium and bone disease in chronic renal failure." *Nephrology, dialysis, transplantation: official publication of the European Dialysis and Transplant Association - European Renal Association* 17 Suppl 2:21-4.

Mjoberg, B., E. Hellquist, H. Mallmin, and U. Lindh. 1997. "Aluminum, Alzheimer's disease and bone fragility." *Acta orthopaedica Scandinavica* 68 (6):511-4.

Shaw, C. A., and L. Tomljenovic. 2013. "Aluminum in the central nervous system (CNS): toxicity in humans and animals, vaccine adjuvants, and autoimmunity." *Immunologic research* 56 (2-3):304-16. doi: 10.1007/s12026-013-8403-1.

Tomljenovic, L. 2011. "Aluminum and Alzheimer's disease: after a century of controversy, is there a plausible link?" *Journal of Alzheimer's disease: JAD* 23 (4):567-98. doi: 10.3233/JAD-2010-101494.

Tomljenovic, L., and C. A. Shaw. 2011. "Aluminum vaccine adjuvants: are they safe?" *Current medicinal chemistry* 18 (17):2630-7.

Wills, M. R., and J. Savory. 1989. "Aluminum and chronic renal failure: sources, absorption, transport, and toxicity." *Critical reviews in clinical laboratory sciences* 27 (1):59-107. doi: 10.3109/10408368909106590

# CHAPTER 4

# Lead

Researchers at the Harvard Medical School have assigned bone lead levels a relative risk factor of 8.8 for cardiovascular disease! This is extraordinarily high; no other risk factor that has been defined in medicine even comes close to this number. Plus, when you consider the trends in cardiovascular disease that seem to come with modern society, it is worth noting that bone lead levels have increased somewhere between 1,000 and 2,000 times in the last 700 years. Nonetheless, a decrease in the environmental presence of lead is often heralded by the Environmental Protection Agency (EPA) as an important success story in the field of environmental health. Once the serious health effects due to lead exposure became unequivocally apparent, the EPA mandated the removal of lead from gasoline and eventually paints and other less apparent sources such as the pencils used by school children (and everyone else). While there has been much progress toward the management of lead in the environment, it still poses a significant health problem for those who become exposed.

## Common Sources for Lead

- Old paint (chips, flakes, houses pre-1975, old toys etc.)
- Contaminated soil (especially around roadways)
- Seafood
- Cosmetics
- Lead pipes (leading to contaminated water)
- Home remedies (Azarcan and Greta)
- Some ceramics and pots
- Some supplements and antacids
- Costume jewelry
- Used car batteries
- Fishing sinkers
- Bullets
- Lead solder
- Stained glass

In addition to cardiovascular disease, lead exposure may cause paralysis and pain in the arms and legs due to its effect on the protective coating that surrounds the nerves and its tendency to cause degeneration of the nervous system. In addition, people who have been exposed to lead may suffer from problems with their vision, hearing, and coordination. Recent research has led to the possibility that lead exposure may increase the risk for dental cavities—an effect that will be continually monitored in the future (Bowen 2001). Lastly, lead exposure is especially dangerous to children—causing serious developmental disorders.

## Common Sources for Lead Exposure

Table 2. Lead within the home (adapted with permission Doctor's Data Inc., 2015).

| Source of Lead | What to Look for |
|---|---|
| **Older Buildings and Homes** | • Lead paint<br>• Tracking lead dust into the home on clothing<br>• Lead dust with home remodeling<br>• Lead pipes and solder |
| **Dust** | • Deteriorating lead paint<br>• Home remodeling creating dust |
| **Soil, Playgrounds and Yards** | • Lead-based paint and other products get into soil<br>• Vegetables in a garden can get contaminated from soil<br>• Exterior fences and paint<br>• Artificial turf on playgrounds |
| **Products** | • Toys and furniture with lead paint<br>• Liquid or food containers<br>• Cosmetics<br>• Plumbing products |
| **Jobs and Hobbies** | • Working with lead, such as strained glass, construction or pottery |

| Drinking Water | • Drinking water coming through lead pipes<br>• Hot water most risky |
|---|---|
| **Folk Remedies** | • Azarcon<br>• Greta<br>• Poto<br>• Nzu<br>• Calabash chalk |

The most common sources for exposure to lead include: drinking water that has travelled through lead pipes, painted toys, some red lipsticks and most cosmetics, lead paint, older homes that still contain lead-based paint, and from the soil around old cars or highways that are contaminated from the days of lead-containing gasoline. Another source for lead exposure that is not highly publicized is through the consumption of fish! While fish containing high levels of mercury have received a lot of public exposure, lead and other heavy metals can also contaminate fish that are living in highly polluted waters (Renieri et al. 2014). Constant vigilance against products that contain lead (and other heavy metals) is necessary to avoid exposure. Lead is continuously found in products that were previously unknown sources of exposure. Just recently, an 18-month old child suffered from severe lead poisoning from an herbal treatment labeled for use in infants and children to treat various cold and flu symptoms (FDA, 2014). The product, known as Bo Ying, is marketed and sold in many retail outlets.

# Lead and the Development of Children

The main concern for children who have been exposed to lead is the severe developmental and cognitive disabilities that may result. This is so well documented that many pediatricians are trained to routinely ask about the possibility of lead exposure for all children, but especially those that seem to be at a higher risk for developmental delays. Children who are suffering from lead exposure typically will show signs of hyperactivity, weight loss, decreased play activity, lower intelligence than their peers, and poor school performance. In children, the most common source of lead exposure is through consumption of lead-based paints that may have been used on toys or flaking paint in older homes. Other possible sources include vegetables that have been grown in lead-contaminated soil, some canned fruit and juices along with evaporated canned milk, or improperly glazed pottery that is used for holding food.

## Lead and the Skeletal System

One of the most insidious consequences of lead poisoning is its ability to take refuge within the bones and cause joint and bone pain as well as osteoporosis leading to fractures. In children, the presence of lead in the bones may result in slowed growth. ***Once lead has deposited itself in the bone, its biological half-life goes from several months to 25-30 years!*** This means that it will take at least 25 years for your body to remove only half of the lead present. It will take another 25 years to remove half of what is left, and so on. You might be tempted to think that it is safer to have lead in your bones than circulating throughout your body—creating all sorts of problems. But, consider this: as your body slowly removes the lead from your bones, it still has to go somewhere. While your body desperately tries to remove this horrendous toxicant, it will pass once again through your entire system as it is taken to your liver and kidneys to be excreted. This means that you will undergo a continual, low-dose exposure until 100 percent of the lead has been removed from the bones, which may be an entire lifetime.

## Lead and the Reproductive System

Lead exposure may diminish fertility rates in both men and women. In men who are exposed over long periods of time, reductions in both the number of sperm as well as their ability to "swim" can occur; also an increase in the number of abnormal sperm is often reported (Alexander et al. 1996). Similarly, in women living near lead smelter facilities an increase in the number of spontaneous abortions, miscarriages, and stillbirths has been reported (McMichael et al. 1986).

## Lead and Kidney Disease

In adults, exposure to lead has been shown to result in lesions on the kidney that may ultimately result in kidney failure, which can have devastating consequences to an individual's quality of life—if not result in death. The damage to the kidney occurs because it is the body's prime mechanism for eliminating lead from the body. As the lead is being flushed through the kidney architecture, it causes significant damage. Then, as the kidney becomes more inflamed, its ability to eliminate lead is also diminished—resulting in greater lead levels throughout the body. Damage to the kidneys as a result of lead poisoning may also lead to chronic illnesses such as hypertension (Kathuria 2013). This is because of the important role that the kidney plays in maintaining fluid levels in the body, which have a direct impact on blood pressure.

## Lead and Blood Disorders

Blood disorders that result from exposure to lead is a secondary effect that is directly related to the amount of kidney damage. Anemia is common in lead poisoning patients. Also, lead interferes with the body's ability to manufacture hemoglobin—the most important oxygen-carrying protein in the body. Without sufficient hemoglobin you will suffer from a lack of oxygen, even though you may be breathing normally.

## Mechanisms of Lead Toxicity

Researchers are continually discovering new information about the ways in which lead causes disease in humans. Some of the best-known pathways include:

- By acting as a potent neurotoxin that results in developmental delays and learning disorders in children and degenerative diseases in adults
- Through its ability to be deposited into the bones, where it avoids removal over many years

- By causing kidney lesions
- By diminishing fertility rates
- By damaging components of the blood, which results in anemia and other disorders

## Key Points about Lead

- Researchers at the Harvard Medical School have assigned bone lead levels a relative risk factor of 8.8 for cardiovascular disease.
- In children, the most common source of lead exposure is through consumption of lead-based paints that may have been used on toys or flaking paint in older homes.
- Once lead has deposited itself in the bone, its biological half-life goes from several months to 25-30 years!

## Chapter 4 References

FDA. 2014. "Bo Ying compound by Eu Yan Sang (Hong Kong) Ltd: FDA/CDER statement--risk of lead poisoning." Drugs.com Accessed October 2, 2014. http://www.drugs.com/fda/bo-ying-compound-eu-yan-sang-hong-kong-ltd-fda-cder-statement-risk-lead-poisoning-13619.html.

Doctor's Data Inc. 2015. Toxic and essential elements.

Alexander, B. H., H. Checkoway, C. van Netten, C. H. Muller, T. G. Ewers, J. D. Kaufman, B. A. Mueller, T. L. Vaughan, and E. M. Faustman. 1996. "Semen quality of men employed at a lead smelter." *Occupational and environmental medicine* 53 (6):411-6.

Bowen, W. H. 2001. "Exposure to metal ions and susceptibility to dental caries." *Journal of dental education* 65 (10):1046-53.

Kathuria, P. 2013. "Lead nephropathy." Accessed September 20, 2014. http://emedicine.medscape.com/article/242605-overview.

McMichael, A. J., G. V. Vimpani, E. F. Robertson, P. A. Baghurst, and P. D. Clark. 1986. "The Port Pirie cohort study: maternal blood lead and pregnancy outcome." *Journal of epidemiology and community health* 40 (1):18-25.

Renieri, E.A., A.K. Alegakis, M. Kiriakakis, M.Vinceti, E. Ozcagli, M.F. Wilks, and A.M. Tsatsakis. 2014. "Cd, Pb and Hg biomonitoring in fish of the Mediterranean region and risk estimations on fish consumption." *Toxics* 2:417-442.

# CHAPTER 5

# Cadmium

Cadmium may not be a heavy metal that you typically worry about at night as you are trying to go to sleep. It does not get the media time that some of the more controversial heavy metals garner, but make no mistake about it: **cadmium is a serious toxicant.** Known as a human carcinogen (which just means it has a proven track record for causing cancer in humans), cadmium damages DNA and prevents the body's DNA repair systems from adequately doing their jobs. The result is cancer. It has also been reported that cadmium "raises special concern because it accumulates in and can damage the kidneys … and it can take 20 years for your body to eliminate even half the cadmium absorbed today" (Mercola 2010). Sound familiar? Longevity within the body is a common theme among many of the heavy metals. Not only that, but cadmium has the disturbing ability to replace zinc in the body. Zinc is an essential mineral that is critical for over 300 enzymatic reactions that occur in the body on a regular basis (International

## Common Sources for Cadmium

- Food sources (shellfish, certain plants such as rice and wheat)
- Tobacco
- Breathing contaminated air
- Zinc, copper, and lead smelter process
- Burning of fossil fuels
- Natural activities (erosion, volcanic activity, river transport)
- Manufacturing of phosphate fertilizers
- Recycling of cadmium steel scrap
- Electric and electronic waste
- Plating material in food processing plants
- Batteries
- Cadmium solder

Zinc Associaton 2011). Zinc is also a critical component for fighting off infections and in fertility. All of that is just to say that Cadmium results in toxicity directly through interactions with DNA and indirectly by interfering with the body's supply of zinc—an incredibly important essential mineral. In addition, cadmium exposure can result in uncomfortable symptoms even at very low levels such as: fever, chills, and muscle aches—sometimes referred to collectively as the "cadmium blues."

## Common Sources for Cadmium Exposure

The most common sources for cadmium exposure are through our food supply, primarily fish (particularly shellfish) and organ meats. Plants are also capable of absorbing cadmium from the soil and water; therefore, occasionally plants grown in particularly contaminated areas can serve as a source of cadmium. Smokers, especially, are at high risk of having an excessively high body burden of cadmium due to the proficiency at which the tobacco plants can uptake cadmium. Exposure can also occur from breathing in contaminated air that is common around industries that burn fossil fuels or municipal waste sites. Cadmium is also a byproduct from the smelter process associated with zinc, copper and lead; therefore, individuals living near these areas tend to have higher than usual levels of cadmium exposure.

## Cadmium and Renal Disease

Chronic renal failure has been reported as endemic in a certain farming region of Sri Lanka. The situation is so dire it has been called "the Trojan horse of the green revolution" (Bandara et al. 2010). Sounds serious, but what could possibly trigger such strong language? It turns out that increases in dietary cadmium due to an agrochemical fertilizer that was added to the farmer's soils in order to boost the production of rice was pinpointed as the cause. Cadmium has repeatedly been implicated in chronic kidney damage and failure, with the effects being accumulative because of the tendency for cadmium to relocate within the kidney tubules once it has been absorbed. Therefore, avoidance of all sources of cadmium exposure and treatment for any current exposures is critical, especially in the presence of other factors that may contribute to kidney disease such as diabetes or hypertension.

## Cadmium and Pulmonary Disorders

There are not many feelings that are worse than an inability to breathe. Cadmium is known to cause changes in lung function, which means that your ability to inhale or exhale may be compromised if you have been exposed to high levels of cadmium. Unfortunately, cadmium is also a common contaminant of cigarette smoke and second hand smoke. Considering the carcinogenic properties of cadmium, it should come as no surprise that cadmium is thought to be one of the main contributors to lung disease—including cancer—in smokers. Not only that, high body burdens of cadmium can as much as double an individual's risk of developing other pulmonary disorders such as emphysema or chronic bronchitis. These are all serious health consequences that can seriously diminish an individual's quality of life. What if you knew that your future included carrying around an oxygen tank, suffering from an inability to breathe, and suffering from any kind of physical exertion? This is the fate shared by many people who are unaware of the high level of cadmium within their body.

## Cadmium and Peripheral Artery Disease

You may be familiar with the term "atherosclerosis" as it applies to the heart and the risk for a heart attack or stroke. Atherosclerosis is a condition of the arteries within the heart in which they become "clogged" by calcium, fat, and cholesterol deposits—commonly known as plaque--that constrict or even block the normal blood flow to the heart, which may result in a heart attack; occasionally, the plaque will become dislodged and result in a stroke. It is less well known that you can develop plaque in the arteries that carry blood to other areas of the body as well; such as your head, various organs, or your arms and legs. When this occurs it is called peripheral artery disease and often results in pain while climbing stairs or simply when walking. The primary risk factor for developing peripheral artery disease is smoking, or more specifically the cadmium found in cigarette smoke.

## Cadmium and the Skeletal System

A common theme observed with many of the toxic heavy metals is their ability to deposit themselves in the bone, which prevents adequate elimination and leads to serious bone disorders such as osteoporosis and bone pain. Cadmium is no exception to this heavy metal trend. It is well documented that cadmium exposure significantly increases the risk for osteoporosis—especially in women and the elderly. However, this process may start at a very early age in children who have been exposed to cadmium (perhaps in the form of second-hand smoke). In fact, in 150 elementary aged school children increases in cadmium levels corresponded with a similar increase in the loss of body calcium levels (Sughis et al. 2011). Clearly, the negative impact of growing children consistently losing significant amounts of calcium is troubling. Unfortunately, as a parent it is important to understand that calcium is an essential mineral for many physiological functions aside from simply bone development. Calcium is also critical for proper muscle function (including the all-important "heart" muscle), cell-to-cell communication, and in neurological processes. Needless to say, seemingly simple exposures to a heavy metal like cadmium can have a negative impact on your health in a variety of ways. Parents: kids are not exempt from the negative health effects of heavy metals!

## Cadmium and Itai-itai Disease

Itai-itai disease is actually the name given to the first documented incident of wide spread cadmium poisoning in the world. The Japanese phrase itai-itai is translated as "ouch-ouch" and the condition was so named because of the painful screams that were common in those who were afflicted. The poisoning cases followed changes in mining practices within the Toyama Prefecture of Japan in which significant amounts of cadmium were released into the nearby Jinzu

River. Victims of itai-itai often suffered conditions of bone softening (osteomalacia) and osteoporosis; at times bone fractures resulted from the force of their body weight alone (Rasnake 2014).

## Cadmium and Cancer

Cadmium is perhaps best known for its known ability to cause cancer. Exposure to cadmium has been linked with numerous types of cancer, including: breast, lung, prostate, kidney, pancreatic, and endometrial cancer. Perhaps the best studied are the links between cadmium and hormone-related cancers such as breast and endometrial cancer. It is hard to imagine, but cadmium can actually "mimic" the physiological effects of estrogen; meaning that cadmium has metalloestrogenic properties (Byrne et al. 2013)!

## Cadmium and Developmental Effects

We know cadmium causes cancer. It accumulates in our bones and kidneys—resulting in a myriad of health problems. It depletes our bodies of calcium. It robs us of our health, but what is it doing to our children? As you might have guessed, *in utero* exposure to cadmium can result in serious developmental deficits in children. In fact, when mothers are exposed to cadmium—and therefore the fetus is exposed to cadmium—the result is decreased birth weights and ultimately decreases in test scores designed to measure intelligence (Tian et al. 2009). Clearly, if you are planning on becoming pregnant, being tested for heavy metals prior to conception is a good idea. If you are already pregnant and suspect you have been exposed, talk with your health care provider about a possible course of action.

## Mechanisms of Cadmium Toxicity

Researchers are continually discovering new information about the ways in which cadmium causes disease in humans. Some of the best-known pathways include:

- By acting as a serious toxicant to the liver and kidneys
- By causing kidney damage; patients often times develop gout as a result, which is an extremely painful condition that often times affects the joints
- By causing loss of systemic calcium reserves—leading to osteomalacia and/or osteoporosis
- By serving as a human carcinogen
- By serving as a "metalloestrogenic" compound

## Key Points about Cadmium

- Cadmium exposure can result in uncomfortable symptoms even at very low levels such as: fever, chills, and muscle aches—sometimes referred to collectively as the "cadmium blues
- Avoidance of all sources of cadmium exposure and treatment for any current exposures is critical, especially in the presence of other factors that may contribute to kidney disease such as diabetes or hypertension
- The primary risk factor for developing peripheral artery disease is smoking, or more specifically the cadmium found in cigarette smoke
- Exposure to cadmium has been linked with numerous types of cancer, including: breast, lung, prostate, kidney, pancreatic, and endometrial cancer

# Chapter 5 References

International Zinc Association. 2011. "Zinc: essential for human health." Accessed September 27, 2014. http://www.zinc.org/info/zinc_essential_for_human_health.

Bandara, J. M., H. V. Wijewardena, J. Liyanege, and M. A. Upul. 2010. "Chronic renal failure in Sri Lanka caused by elevated dietary cadmium: Trojan horse of the green revolution." *Toxicology letters* 198 (1):33-9. doi: 10.1016/j.toxlet.2010.04.016.

Byrne, C., S. D. Divekar, G. B. Storchan, D. A. Parodi, and M. B. Martin. 2013. "Metals and breast cancer." *Journal of mammary gland biology and neoplasia* 18 (1):63-73. doi: 10.1007/s10911-013-9273-9.

Mercola, J. 2010. "Avoid these toxic protein powders until you hear these disturbing details." Accessed September 27, 2014. http://articles.mercola.com/sites/articles/archive/2010/06/22/some-protein-drinks-could-poison-you.aspx.

Rasnake, J. 2014. "Itai-itai disease: a puzzling example of metal toxicity." Accessed September 28, 2014. http://faculty.virginia.edu/metals/cases/rasnake1.html.

Sughis, M., J. Penders, V. Haufroid, B. Nemery, and T. S. Nawrot. 2011. "Bone resorption and environmental exposure to cadmium in children: a cross--sectional study." *Environmental health: a global access science source* 10:104. doi: 10.1186/1476-069X-10-104.

Tian, L. L., Y. C. Zhao, X. C. Wang, J. L. Gu, Z. J. Sun, Y. L. Zhang, and J. X. Wang. 2009. "Effects of gestational cadmium exposure on pregnancy outcome and development in the offspring at age 4.5 years." *Biological trace element research* 132 (1-3):51-9. doi: 10.1007/s12011-009-8391-0.

# CHAPTER 6

# Arsenic

Arsenic--one of the oldest and most notorious of all poisons, is colorless, odorless, tasteless, and a natural component of the environment--characteristics of an ideal poison. Historical cases of arsenic poisoning were notoriously difficult to solve because symptoms could easily be mistaken for food poisoning or other common disorders of the gastrointestinal tract. If the assassin was particularly cautious, arsenic could be given as a series of small doses—resulting in a gradual loss of strength, confusion, and finally paralysis and death.

Today, arsenic is found in the environment both naturally and through anthropogenic activities such as mining, smelting, and coal-fired power plants; arsenic has also been used as a component of pesticides and in the processing of chicken and pigs. While technically a metalloid, arsenic is generally categorized as a heavy metal when discussing its adverse health effects because it shares

> ## Common Sources for Arsenic
>
> - Treated lumber
> - Agricultural products/ pesticides
> - Breathing contaminated air
> - Smelter processes
> - Burning of fossil fuels
> - Contaminated fish
> - Roxarsone-treated chickens
> - Rice grown in areas with high arsenic in the ground and water
> - Fruit juices and some baby foods

many properties that are similar to heavy metals. Chronic arsenic exposure is most typically associated with cancers of the skin, bladder, and lung. Epidemiology evidence also puts arsenic in the category of common risk factors associated with heart disease and peripheral artery diseases.

## Common Sources of Arsenic Exposure

Roughly 70 percent of the arsenic produced worldwide is used for the treatment of lumber, 22 percent is used for agriculture, and the remaining 8 percent is found in glass production, pharmaceutical products, and metallic alloys (Green Facts 2014). Environmental contamination has been a result of metal smelting practices, burning of fossil fuels, arsenic-containing pesticides, and lumber preservation practices. Arsenic can also be found in fish living in highly contaminated waters. Recently, dietary sources of arsenic have raised concern about how much is being consumed in common food sources such as rice. Trace amounts of arsenic have also been found in the meat of chickens treated with an arsenic-containing drug known as Roxarsone. Also, arsenic has been found in alarming concentrations in apple and grape fruit juices as well as jars of baby food such as sweet potatoes, carrots, green beans and peaches (Mercola 2012).

## Arsenic and Cancer

The best-studied outcome following long-term exposure to arsenic is the development of skin cancer--followed by lung, bladder, and kidney cancers. Other skin disorders are commonly reported as well, including hyperkeratosis and pigmentation changes. Generally, high incidences of skin cancer resulting from arsenic exposure occur in areas where the ground water is significantly contaminated. Most of the research has focused on less-developed countries such as Bangladesh, India, and Taiwan; however, alarming concentrations of arsenic in the groundwater have been reported in certain areas of the United States as well. What's more, studies in mice suggest that maternal exposure to arsenic may cause an increase in the susceptibility of her offspring to develop skin cancer (Waalkes et al. 2008). Reports are common for lung and bladder cancers that have developed from drinking arsenic-contaminated water as well as from occupational exposure. Arsenic has a particularly troubling effect on bladder cancer; bladder cancer in arsenic-exposed patients appears to be more aggressive than in people who have no known exposures to arsenic (Moore et al. 2002). Inhaling arsenic in the air as an occupational hazard has a particularly high correlation to levels of lung cancer—the results present an even stronger case when combined with smoking.

## Arsenic and Blackfoot Disease

People living in areas of Taiwan with unusually high levels of arsenic in the groundwater have a high incidence of a severe form of peripheral vascular disease often called "Blackfoot disease." In the case of Blackfoot disease, the loss of circulation is so severe that the patient will often times develop gangrene and become at risk for limb amputations. This has serious implications when considering the demonstrated link between low levels of arsenic exposure and the increased risk of cardiovascular disease. The implication is that the low(er) levels of arsenic in the drinking water that are more typically observed in the United States could result in equally devastating effects to the cardiovascular system as a whole—and may be a significant contributor to the incidence of hypertension and other cardiovascular diseases. Evidence does, in fact, support this idea.

## Arsenic and Cardiovascular Disease

Epidemiology has repeatedly suggested that there is a positive relationship between arsenic exposure and vascular disease, particularly atherosclerosis (Simeonova and Luster 2004). It is very likely that arsenic increases heart disease through the formation of free radicals and an increase in oxidative stress (Wu et al. 2003). It is a well-known fact that heart disease is the number one killer of both men and women. This results in a huge cost, both in monetary terms and quality of life value. Considering the widespread presence of arsenic in ground water across the U.S., it is not a difficult stretch to connect the dots. Future avoidance of arsenic and appropriate treatment measures following any type of exposure might just prevent a future episode of open-heart surgery.

## Mechanisms of Arsenic Toxicity

Researchers are continually discovering new information about the ways in which arsenic causes disease in humans. Some of the best-known pathways include:

- Causing genetic abnormalities that contribute to the risk of cancer
- Increasing the formation of free radicals resulting in increased oxidative stress
- Causing chronic vasoconstriction resulting in an increased risk for heart disease

## Key Points about Arsenic

- Chronic arsenic exposure is most typically associated with cancers of the skin, bladder, and lung.
- Epidemiology evidence puts arsenic in the category of common risk factors associated with heart disease and peripheral artery diseases
- Epidemiology has repeatedly suggested that there is a positive relationship between arsenic exposure and vascular disease, particularly atherosclerosis

## Chapter 6 References

Green Facts. 2014. "Arsenic." Accessed October 4, 2014. http://www. greenfacts.org/en/arsenic/l-3/arsenic-1.htm - 0p0.

Mercola, J. 2012. "Dr. Oz proves this fruit juice can be toxic." Accessed October 4, 2014. http://articles.mercola.com/sites/articles/ archive/2012/01/22/toxic-metals-on-fruit-juices.aspx.

Moore, L. E., A. H. Smith, C. Eng, D. Kalman, S. DeVries, V. Bhargava, K. Chew, D. Moore, 2nd, C. Ferreccio, O. A. Rey, and F. M. Waldman. 2002. "Arsenic-related chromosomal alterations in bladder cancer." *Journal of the National Cancer Institute* 94 (22):1688-96.

Simeonova, P. P., and M. I. Luster. 2004. "Arsenic and atherosclerosis." *Toxicology and applied pharmacology* 198 (3):444-9. doi: 10.1016/j. taap.2003.10.018.

Waalkes, M. P., J. Liu, D. R. Germolec, C. S. Trempus, R. E. Cannon, E. J. Tokar, R. W. Tennant, J. M. Ward, and B. A. Diwan. 2008. "Arsenic exposure in utero exacerbates skin cancer response in adulthood with contemporaneous distortion of tumor stem cell dynamics." *Cancer research* 68 (20):8278-85. doi: 10.1158/0008-5472.CAN-08-2099.

Wu, M. M., H. Y. Chiou, I. C. Ho, C. J. Chen, and T. C. Lee. 2003. "Gene expression of inflammatory molecules in circulating lymphocytes from arsenic-exposed human subjects." *Environmental health perspectives* 111 (11):1429-38.

# CHAPTER 7

# Iron

Considering the role that iron plays in your health, iron toxicity can be a confusing issue; iron is both an essential element for life and highly toxic to our bodies. This makes navigating the complicated issue of iron levels in our body difficult. Forming and maintaining a positive relationship with a health care provider who specializes in heavy metals will be instrumental in ensuring that your iron levels are properly balanced.

Iron is a key component of hemoglobin, the life-giving protein that circulates in your blood and delivers oxygen from your lungs to the rest of your tissues. It also serves as a critical component of many enzymes that help to maintain normal body functions as well as playing a role in cell growth and differentiation. However, iron is also an extremely reactive metal that loves to be involved in unhealthy reactions that result in extreme oxidative stress. For this reason, iron is tightly regulated and heavily "safe-guarded" in your body to prevent these toxic properties from making you sick instead of giving you life. In fact, your body produces an important protein called ferritin that has the important job of sequestering iron and holding it in a form that prevents it from causing damage to your cells and tissues. However, at some point, the iron levels circulating in your body may exceed the body's ability to regulate them—resulting in an increased risk for things such as cancer and cardiovascular disease. Increases in the free radicals associated with iron overload and oxidative stress is also a catalyst for rapid aging!

## Common Sources of Iron

Common sources of excess iron in the diet include the use of iron pots or pans for cooking, particularly if you are cooking very acidic foods. Processed food is another common source for excess iron. A high percentage of processed foods are "iron fortified" and often times the iron added to these products is inorganic iron, which is a much more dangerous form than the organic iron that comes from meat and other natural sources. Well water is another common source for increased iron intake. Under normal conditions, the oxygen in the air will oxidize iron in the water—causing it to precipitate out and settle to the bottom, which reduces the amount of iron present in the water. However, well water is not typically exposed to a sufficient amount of oxygen to convert the iron from its reduced and water soluble form, to its oxidized and water insoluble form. Vitamin and mineral supplements present another route that might contribute to iron overload as many of these supplements contain iron. Finally, regular consumption of alcohol may increase your absorption of iron and contribute to iron overload (Mercola 2013).

## Hemochromatosis

Hemochromatosis is the technical term used to describe a condition of iron overload. Because iron is an essential component for life, your body lacks any efficient mechanism for removing excess amounts. As a result, it accumulates in the body and becomes toxic to your cells, tissues, and organs (Ramm and Ruddell 2010).

There are two types of hemochromatosis: a hereditary form that is passed down from parents to offspring, and a secondary type that is usually due to outside conditions such as anemia or liver disease. Symptoms are often times very generic and include things like joint pain, fatigue, and stomach pain. Without treatment, iron may build up in the organs and result in liver damage, as well as complications for diabetes, arrhythmias, arthritis, and erectile dysfunction.

## Cardiovascular disease

High levels of oxidative stress are thought to be one of the primary conditions that increase an individual's risk for heart disease. Iron overload is a huge source of free radicals and oxidative stress. These free radicals react with circulating fatty acids and other lipids in the blood—changing them into a form that is no longer beneficial for one's health. These altered lipids then contribute to the formation of atherosclerotic plaque that builds up in the arteries and peripheral vasculature and eventually may cause a heart attack, stroke, or other type of cardiovascular disease. A study conducted in Finland on over 2,000 individuals showed that levels of stored iron within the

**Common Sources for Iron**

- Cooking with iron pots and pans
- Eating "iron fortified" processed foods
- Well water containing high levels of iron
- Drinking alcohol along with high iron-containing foods

body was a better predictor for heart attack risk than either high blood pressure or cholesterol (Walling 2011)! Similarly, other studies have shown that reducing your body's iron burden can reduce your risk of suffering from a heart attack or stroke (Zacharski, Shamayeva, and Chow 2011).

In addition to clearly defined cardiovascular diseases, iron is known to contribute to a condition that is known as metabolic syndrome (Abril-Ulloa et al. 2014). Metabolic syndrome is diagnosed in patients who exhibit a series of conditions that when combined, present an overall increase in the risk of heart disease, stroke, and diabetes. If you have been diagnosed with increased blood pressure, high blood sugar levels, excess abdominal fat, and abnormal cholesterol—you may have metabolic syndrome and should have your body iron levels checked to prevent exacerbating the condition further.

## Cancer

It has long been known that a high body burden of iron poses a significant risk for the development of liver cancer. More recently, epidemiology has suggested that excessive levels of iron in the body may also contribute to colorectal, colon, breast, and lung cancer (Fonseca-Nunes, Jakszyn, and Agudo 2014)! The positive correlation between high body levels of iron and the various forms of cancer is most likely due to the high oxidative potential (and free radical formation) that is characteristic of iron. You can liken this phenomenon of iron in the body to what happens to iron metals when they have been left outside in the elements—but instead of rust, iron is damaging the DNA, proteins, and lipids within the body resulting in cancer and other adverse health effects.

## Diabetes

There are two main types of diabetes: type 1 and type 2. Type 1 diabetes is an autoimmune disease that affects the body's ability to synthesize insulin and therefore regulate blood sugar levels. These patients require regular monitoring of their blood sugar levels and self-administration of an exogenous source of insulin in order to keep normal sugar levels in the blood. Type 2 diabetics, on the other hand, still produce insulin, but their body has lost its ability to respond to it in an appropriate fashion—a condition known as insulin resistance. As the body loses its ability to manage the glucose, it builds up in the blood and causes extensive damage throughout the body. The extent of protective mechanisms that biological systems employ in order to regulate various molecules in the body can give you an idea of their toxic potential when imbalances occur. Sugar is a great example. Sugar levels within the blood are very tightly regulated through a complex system of checks and balances. Sugar is primarily responsible for all of the health complications that are frequently seen in diabetic patients. Needless to say, it is a risk for type 2 diabetes that has been shown to increase in people with excessively high iron levels in the body, an affect that is increasingly gaining attention (Zhao et al. 2012). It is interesting to note that frequent blood donations are associated with increased sensitivity to insulin and a decrease in the incidence of type 2 diabetes.

# Liver Disease (Cirrhosis)

Liver cirrhosis is a chronic inflammatory condition that results in a buildup of scar tissue on the liver that prevents this vital organ from functioning at full capacity. Among relatively young adults (aged 30-50) liver cirrhosis is the fourth most common cause of death. The role that iron plays in liver disease, particularly alcoholic cirrhosis, is so devastating that researchers have actually been able to predict the likelihood for death in patients based on their liver iron levels (Ganne-Carrie et al. 2000). While this should be "sobering" news for alcoholics, it also has relevance for social drinkers as well. It has been shown that alcohol consumption increases the bioavailability of iron from common food sources. Considering the wide array of toxicants that we are continually exposed to and the fact that our liver is arguably one of the most important organs for "detoxing," the influence of even social drinking on our body iron levels bears consideration.

# Mechanisms of Iron Toxicity

Researchers are continually discovering new information about the ways in which iron causes disease in humans. Some of the best-known pathways include:

- As an extremely reactive compound with high oxidizing potential, iron is a huge source of free radical generation and oxidative stress
- As a carcinogen
- As a liver and heart toxicant
- By decreasing the body's sensitivity to insulin

# Key Points about Iron

- Iron is a key component of hemoglobin, the life-giving protein that circulates in your blood and delivers oxygen from your lungs to the rest of your tissues

- Increases in the free radicals associated with iron overload and oxidative stress is also a catalyst for rapid aging
- A high body burden of iron poses a significant risk for the development of liver cancer
- The role that iron plays in liver disease, particularly alcoholic cirrhosis, is so devastating that researchers have actually been able to predict the likelihood for death in patients based on their liver iron levels

# Chapter 7 References

Abril-Ulloa, V., G. Flores-Mateo, R. Sola-Alberich, B. Manuel-y-Keenoy, and V. Arija. 2014. "Ferritin levels and risk of metabolic syndrome: meta-analysis of observational studies." *BMC public health* 14:483. doi: 10.1186/1471-2458-14-483.

Fonseca-Nunes, A., P. Jakszyn, and A. Agudo. 2014. "Iron and cancer risk--a systematic review and meta-analysis of the epidemiological evidence." *Cancer epidemiology, biomarkers & prevention: a publication of the American Association for Cancer Research, cosponsored by the American Society of Preventive Oncology* 23 (1):12-31. doi: 10.1158/1055-9965.EPI-13-0733.

Ganne-Carrie, N., C. Christidis, C. Chastang, M. Ziol, F. Chapel, F. Imbert-Bismut, J. C. Trinchet, C. Guettier, and M. Beaugrand. 2000. "Liver iron is predictive of death in alcoholic cirrhosis: a multivariate study of 229 consecutive patients with alcoholic and/or hepatitis C virus cirrhosis: a prospective follow up study." *Gut* 46 (2):277-82.

Mercola, J. 2013. "Iron in your blood." Accessed October 11, 2014. http://articles.mercola.com/sites/articles/archive/2013/06/05/elevated-iron-levels.aspx.

Ramm, G. A., and R. G. Ruddell. 2010. "Iron homeostasis, hepatocellular injury, and fibrogenesis in hemochromatosis: the role of inflammation in a noninflammatory liver disease." *Seminars in liver disease* 30 (3):271-87. doi: 10.1055/s-0030-1255356.

Walling, E. 2011. "Iron supplements cause more harm than good." *Natural News*, Monday, October 31, 2011.

Zacharski, L. R., G. Shamayeva, and B. K. Chow. 2011. "Effect of controlled reduction of body iron stores on clinical outcomes in peripheral arterial disease." *American heart journal* 162 (5):949-957 e1. doi: 10.1016/j.ahj.2011.08.013.

Zhao, Z., S. Li, G. Liu, F. Yan, X. Ma, Z. Huang, and H. Tian. 2012. "Body iron stores and heme-iron intake in relation to risk of type 2 diabetes: a systematic review and meta-analysis." *PloS one* 7 (7):e41641. doi: 10.1371/journal.pone.0041641.

# CHAPTER 8

# Copper

Along with iron, copper is an essential nutrient that is necessary to maintain life. Copper plays a critical function in the body's natural defenses against oxidative stress as a component of an enzyme called *superoxide dismutase* or SOD. SOD is a natural antioxidant that is produced by the body in order to defuse the reactive nature of free radicals that are constantly being produced as a natural byproduct of energy production and from exposure to a myriad of environmental toxicants. However, like all metals—including the essential metals, overexposure or imbalances will result in adverse health effects.

The average American consuming a western diet exceeds the daily nutritional requirements

## Common Sources for Copper

- Copper cookware
- Birth control and copper intrauterine devices
- Well water containing high levels of copper
- Vitamin and mineral supplements
- Fungicides from swimming pools and food
- Vegetarian and other high copper diets
- Occupational exposure
- Dental alloys in fillings
- Adrenal gland exhaustion
- Zinc deficiency

for copper. Elevated levels of copper in the body can result in "paranoid and hallucinatory schizophrenia, hypertension, preeclampsia, stuttering, autism, childhood hyperactivity, premenstrual tensions, psychiatric depression, insomnia, senility and possibly functional hypoglycemia" (Pfeiffer 1975).

## Common Sources of Copper

Copper is commonly used to control the growth of various organisms including bacterial, fungal, and aquatic species. Because of this property, copper is commonly included in mouthwashes and toothpaste to control bacteria and plaque formation. Copper is also extensively used in fish farming to control the growth of unwanted aquatic organisms. In addition, birth control devices, particularly copper containing intrauterine devices can be a significant source of extraneous copper in women along with leaching from copper-containing cookware. High copper levels can be found in some water supplies and diets that include a high percentage of foods with significant amounts of copper, such as soybeans, nuts, seeds, tofu, avocados and grains can increase the risk of copper overload. Occupational exposure can sometimes be a problem for professionals working in the plumbing, welding and machine industries as well.

There are also several pathological conditions that can contribute to excessive body copper levels in the absence of an outside exposure. Adrenal exhaustion, for example, can result in diminished production of the protein ceruloplasmin that is necessary for "carrying" copper throughout the body. When levels of ceruloplasmin decline, then levels of "free" copper increase in the body, which allows copper to accumulate in various tissues and organs. Zinc deficiency is another pathological condition that contributes to copper overload. Zinc and copper work to maintain a delicate balance in the body—deficiencies in one can lead to excessive concentrations of the other. It is much more common for people to be deficient in zinc than in copper.

## Cancer

Copper serves a vital role in the regulation of cell growth. Cancer is, by definition, a loss of cell growth regulation. That's why a recent article, entitled "copper intake makes tumors breathe" may say it all (Lausanne 2013). While researchers do not necessarily believe that copper causes cancer (although it might), copper does make it easier for cancer cells to proliferate, or grow. Because of their extremely high growth rate, cancer cells require excessive amounts of energy. Copper, as a critical component of many energy-producing enzymes, can help provide cancer cells with the energy they need. A similar headline: "Bad penny: Cancer's thirst for copper can be targeted," suggests that prevention of copper absorption may be a viable treatment option for some types of cancer (Medicine 2014). That is certainly food for thought. At the very least, awareness of your current copper status may keep you from inadvertently assisting possible tumor growth.

## Alzheimer's Disease

A recent study reported an increased risk of Alzheimer's disease following low doses of copper in the drinking water of mice (Singh et al. 2013). It is thought that copper may contribute to the onset of Alzheimer's disease by preventing the brain from clearing out toxic compounds by breaking down the blood brain barrier. Researchers noted, "that the copper stimulated activity in neurons increased the production of amyloid beta. The copper also interacted with amyloid beta in a manner that caused the proteins to bind together in larger complexes creating logjams of the protein that the brain's waste disposal system cannot clear" (Redorbit 2013). It is clear that unhealthy levels of copper in the system has a negative impact on the blood brain barrier—the brain's first line of defense against toxic compounds.

## Wilson's Disease

Wilson's disease is an inherited disease that affects copper metabolism and the body's ability to clear copper from the system. While Wilson's disease is relatively rare (1 in 30,000 people are diagnosed), it is a very severe condition (Rosencrantz 2011). According to the Mayo Clinic, individuals with Wilson's disease may experience the following symptoms (Mayo Clinic 2014):

- Fatigue, lack of appetite or abdominal pain
- Jaundice, a yellowing of the skin and the whites of the eye

- A tendency to bruise easily
- Fluid buildup in the legs or abdomen
- Problems with speech, swallowing or physical coordination
- Uncontrolled movements or muscle stiffness

Uncontrolled Wilson's disease may result in severe liver damage and must be properly managed. Chelation therapy is one viable option. Please talk with your health care provider immediately if you suspect that you have Wilson's disease.

## Mechanisms of Copper Toxicity

Researchers are continually discovering new information about the ways in which copper causes disease in humans. Some of the best-known pathways include:

- Providing cancer cells with energy
- Depleting the body of zinc
- As a liver toxicant
- By inhibiting the clearance of amyloid plaques—contributing to Alzheimer's disease
- By damaging the blood brain barrier and contributing to neuro-inflammation
- By producing free radicals and contributing to oxidative stress

## Key Points about Copper

- Elevated levels of copper in the body can result in paranoid and hallucinatory schizophrenia, hypertension, preeclampsia, stuttering, autism, childhood hyperactivity, premenstrual tensions, psychiatric depression, insomnia, senility and possibly functional hypoglycemia
- Zinc deficiency is another pathological condition that contributes to copper overload.

- Zinc and copper work to maintain a delicate balance in the body—deficiencies in one can lead to excessive concentrations of the other
- Wilson's disease is an inherited disease that affects copper metabolism and the body's ability to clear copper from the system. Uncontrolled Wilson's disease may result in severe liver damage and must be properly managed

# Chapter 8 References

Redorbit. 2013. "Copper found to play a role in onset, progression of Alzheimer's disease." Accessed October 12, 2014. http://www.redorbit.com/news/health/1112926979/alzheimers-disease-linked-to-too-much-copper-082013/.

Mayo Clinic. 2014. "Wilson's disease: symptoms." Accessed October 12, 2014. http://www.mayoclinic.org/diseases-conditions/wilsons-disease/basics/symptoms/con-20043499.

Lausanne, Ecole Polytechnique Federale de. 2013. "Copper intake makes tumors breathe." Accessed October 12, 2104. http://www.sciencedaily.com/releases/2013/11/131114102526.htm.

Medicine, Duke. 2014. "Bad penny: cancer's thirst for copper can be targeted." Accessed October 12, 2014. http://www.sciencedaily.com/releases/2014/04/140409134310.htm.

Pfeiffer, C.C. 1975. *Mental and elemental nutrients*: Keats Publishing.

Rosencrantz, R.R. 2011. "Wilson disease: pathogenesis and clinical considerations in diagnosis and treatment." *Seminars in liver disease* 31 (3):245-259.

Singh, I., A. P. Sagare, M. Coma, D. Perlmutter, R. Gelein, R. D. Bell, R. J. Deane, E. Zhong, M. Parisi, J. Ciszewski, R. T. Kasper, and R. Deane. 2013. "Low levels of copper disrupt brain amyloid-beta homeostasis by altering its production and clearance." *Proceedings of the National Academy of Sciences of the United States of America* 110 (36):14771-6. doi: 10.1073/pnas.1302212110.

# CHAPTER 9

# Thallium

Thallium is an extremely toxic metal to humans—more so even than mercury, cadmium and lead. Since its discovery in 1861 it has been involved in many poisoning cases, both accidental and deliberate. Thallium resembles the chemical makeup of potassium and as a consequence can disrupt many of the potassium-dependent pathways and processes within the body. Potassium is an electrolyte that is important in the body in order for muscles to contract—including the heart. Imbalances in potassium levels can have immediate and life threatening consequences. In addition, exposure to thallium typically results in gastrointestinal disturbances, neurological disorders, disruption of calcium homeostasis, and hair loss (Mulkey and Oehme 1993). Historically, thallium was used to treat a variety of illnesses, including syphilis, gonorrhea, tuberculosis, and ringworm. Unfortunately, a thallium-containing product known as Koremlu resulted in 692 cases of thallium poisoning and numerous deaths within the United States shortly after entering the market as a depilatory (hair removal) agent. In 1932, various headlines reported on the issue with titles such as: "another case of thallium poisoning following use of Koremlu cream"; "Koremlu cream—a disclaimer"; and "case study: thallium poisoning." At the time, thallium was also used as a rodent and ant killer, which remained in effect until 1965 when it was finally banned following multiple poisonings (Rusyniak, Furbee, and Kirk 2002). Thallium has also been a popular poison used for criminal activities due to its odorless and tasteless properties. Currently, thallium is not produced within the United States; however, it is imported for use in the manufacture of various commercial products including electronics, thermometers, and jewelry.

Victims of thallium exposure will experience severe nausea, vomiting and diarrhea and nervous system damage within the first 72 hours. The neurotoxic effects result in pain, reduced reflexes, convulsions, loss of muscle tone, headaches, numbness, symptoms of dementia, and occasionally coma. Within two weeks after exposure, the characteristic signs of hair loss (alopecia) are seen; within three weeks heart disturbances become evident.

## Common Sources of Thallium

In the environment, thallium exists as a rare element that is found in the Earth's crust and to a certain extent in the air. Thallium is water-soluble and therefore can easily contaminate water supplies. Similarly, thallium can easily be taken up into plant crops and enter

### Common Sources for Thallium

- Eating contaminated food
- Industrial exposures
- Smoking
- Living near hazardous waste sites
- Incidental ingestion of contaminated soil or water
- Breathing contaminated air from coal-burning and smelting processes
- Through some medical imaging procedures
- Rodent poisons

the food chain through agricultural practices. Thallium is also used in some medical imaging procedures. Unfortunately, conventional methods for removing heavy metals from water supplies are ineffective against thallium (Peter and Viraraghavan 2005).

## Neurological Effects

The most devastating consequences of thallium exposure are the short- and long-term neurological effects. Exposure can cause mild to severe neurological damage leading to comas and even death. Unfortunately, excessive neurological deficits often occur because doctors are unable to make a quick diagnosis. Often times, patients who have been acutely exposed do not start showing the "hallmark symptom" for thallium exposure (hair loss) until several weeks after the initial exposure has occurred. Generally, by this time the damage is so extensive that patients do not always fully recover.

# Alopecia

Alopecia is a term that is used to describe extensive hair loss from some or all areas of the body. This is a "hallmark" symptom of thallium poisoning and, in fact, thallium has been marketed as a depilatory agent—with severe consequences. Currently, thallium poisoning will be a primary consideration in medical conditions that are otherwise difficult to diagnose but include alopecia as a symptom.

# Mechanisms of Thallium Toxicity

Researchers are continually discovering new information about the ways in which thallium causes disease in humans. Some of the best-known pathways include:

- Competing with the body's stores of potassium
- Inhibiting DNA synthesis
- Causing neurological damage
- Alopecia
- Kidney failure

# Key Points about Thallium

- Thallium resembles the chemical makeup of potassium and as a consequence can disrupt many of the potassium-dependent pathways and processes within the body
- A thallium-containing product known as Koremlu resulted in 692 cases of thallium poisoning and numerous deaths within the United States shortly after entering the market as a depilatory (hair removal) agent

# Chapter 9 References

Mulkey, J. P., and F. W. Oehme. 1993. "A review of thallium toxicity." *Veterinary and human toxicology* 35 (5):445-53.

Peter, A. L., and T. Viraraghavan. 2005. "Thallium: a review of public health and environmental concerns." *Environment international* 31 (4):493-501. doi: 10.1016/j.envint.2004.09.003.

Rusyniak, D. E., R. B. Furbee, and M. A. Kirk. 2002. "Thallium and arsenic poisoning in a small midwestern town." *Annals of emergency medicine* 39 (3):307-11.

# CHAPTER 10

# Nickel

Nickel is another example of a heavy metal that most people would not consider to be a worrisome factor toward achieving optimal health. Many people wear nickel-containing jewelry or own nickel-plated mirrors or other decorative items. However, the truth is that nickel presents a significant hazard to your health. In addition to being a carcinogen, chronic exposure to nickel may also contribute to "cardiovascular disease, neurological deficits, developmental deficits in childhood, and high blood pressure" (Chervona, Arita, and Costa 2012).

## Sources

Because nickel is such a versatile metal, it is commonly used in a variety of common household items. Stainless steel cookware may contain as much as 14 percent nickel, similarly, costume jewelry often contains very high levels of nickel. Nickel is also released into the atmosphere by catalytic converters found in automobiles. It is also very worrisome to consider that nickel is a very efficient "catalyst" for use in a variety of reactions, from the process used to hydrogenate the fats found in margarine to the production of high-tech medical

### Common Sources for Nickel

- Orthodontic hardware
- Jewelry
- Occupational exposures
- Common household items such as nickel-plated mirrors
- As a component of coins, magnets, electronics, and stainless steel
- As a common contaminant of "engineered nanomaterials" found in sunscreens, other medical applications, and many other industrial uses

devices utilizing engineered nanomaterials. As a consequence, many of these items are contaminated with trace levels of nickel—presenting a significant source of exposure. What's more, as nickel is increasingly used in the manufacture of high-tech devices, its presence as a contaminant in the environment will continually be on the rise.

## Contact Dermatitis

Contact dermatitis is the most common side effect associated with nickel exposure. Caused by an allergic reaction to nickel, contact dermatitis is an itchy rash that results from any dermal (skin) contact with nickel. Once an individual develops contact dermatitis from nickel, subsequent exposures may result in increasingly severe cases of irritation. Approximately 10–20 percent of the general population develops contact dermatitis after nickel exposure.

## Summary of Adverse Effects from Nickel Exposure

Aside from contact dermatitis, exposure to nickel has reportedly caused adverse effects to the respiratory tract following inhalation exposure, to the immune system following inhalation, oral, or dermal exposure, and possibly the reproductive system and the developing offspring following oral exposure (Center for Disease Control 2014).

## Mechanisms of Nickel Toxicity

Researchers are continually discovering new information about the ways in which nickel causes disease in humans. Some of the best-known pathways include:

- As a human carcinogen
- Through the formation of free radicals and oxidative stress
- By causing an increase in inflammation
- By disrupting the balance of essential minerals

## Key Points about Nickel

- In addition to being a carcinogen, chronic exposure to nickel may also contribute to cardiovascular disease, neurological deficits, developmental deficits in childhood, and high blood pressure
- Approximately 10–20 percent of the general population develops contact dermatitis after nickel exposure
- As nickel is increasingly used in the manufacture of high-tech devices, its presence as a contaminant in the environment will continually be on the rise

# Chapter 10 References

Center for Disease Control. 2014. "Toxicological profile for nickel." Accessed October 18, 2014. http://www.atsdr.cdc.gov/toxprofiles/tp15-c2.pdf.

Chervona, Y., A. Arita, and M. Costa. 2012. "Carcinogenic metals and the epigenome: understanding the effect of nickel, arsenic, and chromium." *Metallomics: integrated biometal science* 4 (7):619-27. doi: 10.1039/c2mt20033c.

# CHAPTER 11

# Exposure to Multiple Heavy Metals

If you are still not convinced that exposure to heavy metals applies to you, then consider that most people are not exposed to just one heavy metal, but rather multiple heavy metals at different times and in different ways throughout their lifetime. Why is that important? ***Exposure to more than one heavy metal creates a kind of "toxic synergy" between the two compounds that does not bode well for your health.*** Take, for example, an experiment that was conducted in rats that were exposed to low levels of mercury or aluminum. The unfortunate rats suffered a mortality rate of approximately 1 in 100 following exposure. However, when the rats were exposed to mercury and aluminum *at the same time*, 100 percent of them died (Haley 2007). Think about this for a minute. The same dose of each heavy metal was given in each experiment, but when they were administered together the toxicity of BOTH metals was exponentially increased! Still not convinced this applies to you? Ask yourself this or a similar question: Have you ever cooked a tuna steak in aluminum foil? Chances are that you were exposed to a dose of mercury from the fish and aluminum that leached from the foil—at the same time. Thus some of these toxicants stay in your system and over the years, the more exposure you have, the more they build up in your system!

The many ways in which an exposure to one metal can impact the response of the body to other environmental toxicants is one of the most frightening aspects of heavy metal toxicity. Take, for example, the relationship between cadmium and zinc within the body. The body is easily fooled into "up taking" cadmium in the place of zinc in very large quantities. To make it worse, normal signaling mechanisms that tell the body to stop absorbing zinc do not function in the presence of cadmium—resulting in continual and un-checked absorption of cadmium as long as there is a source of exposure (Rasnake 2014).

Here are other common interactions that you should know about:

- Alcohol consumption tends to increase the absorption of iron, which may result in iron overload.
- Fluoride has been shown to increase the absorption of lead and compete with iodide—a necessary component for proper thyroid functions.
- Co-exposures of copper and excess iron can also compound the toxicity of both metals.
- Copper is also known to adversely affect the body stores of zinc.
- Fluoride and excessive phosphorus can decrease the absorption of calcium.
- Lead, cadmium, sodium, potassium and high protein diets all increase the loss of calcium in the urine.
- Chromium absorption can be inhibited by the presence of iron, manganese, zinc, vanadium and phytates (typically found in whole grains, nuts and seeds).
- Molybdenum binds copper and is therefore considered to be a powerful copper antagonist.
- Molybdenum can remove copper from the body without affecting zinc levels, making it a powerful tool for helping with copper overload.
- Molybdenum intake raises sodium levels.
- Molybdenum absorption is inhibited in the presence of copper, sulfur and methionine.
- The body cannot adequately metabolize molybdenum in the presence of manganese, zinc and sulfur.
- Calcium, iron, phosphorus, and soy protein all inhibit the absorption of molybdenum.
- Absorption of phosphorus can be inhibited in the presence of aluminum, calcium, iron, magnesium and vitamin D deficiency.
- Several metals antagonize the proper functions of zinc, including cadmium, chromium, copper, iron, manganese and selenium.

## Chapter 11 References

Haley, B.E. 2007. "The relationship of the toxic effects of mercury to exacerbation of the medical condition classified as Alzheimer's disease." *Medical Veritas* 4:1510–1524.

Rasnake, J. 2014. "Itai–itai disease: a puzzling example of metal toxicity." Accessed September 28, 2014. http://faculty.virginia.edu/metals/cases/rasnake1.html.

# CHAPTER 12

# A 6-Step Program to Overcoming Heavy Metal Exposure-Overview

"There is a predictable way that the body breaks down. It doesn't happen in different ways in different people ... There's a methodical way you can test and correct all these issues." Overcoming significant heavy metal exposures can seem like a daunting task. Luckily, with the information presented in this book, along with a little perseverance and time, you will very quickly be on the path toward improved health and well-being! This chapter will give you a brief outline of 6 critical steps that you should follow in your journey toward being free of the symptoms of heavy metal toxicity.

> "There is a predictable way that the body breaks down. It doesn't happen in different ways in different people ... There's a methodical way you can test and correct all these issues."
>
> -Dr. Daniel Kalish (Founder of "The Kalish Method" & Author of *Mind Mapping*)

## 1. Get Tested!

Establishing a baseline for your individual burden of heavy metals will provide you with information that will: 1) help you tailor a recovery program that is specific for your own particular needs, 2) provide a marker by which you can gauge your progress toward becoming free of the burdens of heavy metals and 3) provide you with information about the heavy metals in your environment that are particularly troublesome and should be eliminated if at all possible.

There are various types of tests that can be used for measuring your particular burden of heavy metals. These include analyzing samples from whole blood, red blood cells, serum, urine, fecal matter and hair. Each of these tests is discussed in more detail in Chapter 14.

There is also a list of resources at the end of the book that can be used to locate practitioners in your area that can help you in your journey. You can also visit my website at: www.drpamelaowens.com or www.drpamowens.com/blog and order a test (unless restricted in your area: including NY, NJ and RI) that will entitle you to a personal evaluation of your results along with recommendations on how to proceed with your treatment.

## 2. Get Treated!

As they say, **knowledge is power!** Once you know exactly what your unique profile of heavy metal exposures looks like, you and your health care provider can easily choose a treatment plan that will specifically address the heavy metals that are troublesome for you and your unique situation. Chelation therapy is the standard practice for removing heavy metal exposure and can be done through intravenous infusions or by taking oral supplements. Each has its own advantages and should be considered carefully based on your results from the heavy metals testing. Additional information on the benefits and details of chelation therapy is given in Chapter 15. A list of additional resources is also provided at the end of the book.

It is especially important that you undergo chelation therapy with the assistance of a knowledgeable health care provider who specializes in heavy metals toxicity and has been trained in the procedures necessary for ensuring that your experience is beneficial and without risk. Regardless, chelation therapy has been proven to be an extremely safe treatment for the vast majority of patients.

## 3. Remove and Avoid Sources of Exposure

The presence of heavy metals and other toxicants surround us. This is our modern day reality, but that does not mean we are helpless in our efforts to find good health. Learning about the most common sources for exposure and minimizing them will go a long way toward reducing the burden of heavy metals on your health. In addition, vigilant monitoring (see step # 1) will enable you to detect any time you may have inadvertently been exposed to heavy metals and give you the opportunity to be treated and to remove the source of exposure. For more information, please see details provided in Chapter 16.

## 4. Boost Your Natural Detoxification Systems

We all have a built in system for detoxifying toxic compounds, whether they are produced internally or if we are exposed to them through external sources. This is great news! The detoxification pathways are broken down into two distinct phases, known as Phase I and Phase II, but we'll talk more about their differences in Chapter 17. For now, it is important to understand that in order to properly take care of your body, the detox pathways require a support system that you are responsible for providing! In particular, detoxification pathways rely on a properly balanced diet that provides the appropriate ratio of fats, fiber, minerals, protein, phytochemicals and vitamins. Finally, remember that like any system, it is possible to overwhelm your detoxification pathways with a constant burden of toxic substances. That's why it is so important that you take the initiative to remove as many of these as possible from your surroundings and minimize your exposure whenever (and wherever!) you can.

## 5. Boost Your Overall Health

Steps number four and five in my heavy metals detox plan are very similar in that if you boost your natural detoxification pathways, you will also boost your overall health and some of the methods are the same. But, there are also things that you can do that will improve your health and well-being apart from your internal detox machinery.

One of the most important steps you can take is to make a commitment to eating only foods that have been designated as "organic" by the USDA whenever possible. I understand that there are often budget limitations to buying foods organic, which is why I recommend you familiarize yourself with the information provided by the Environmental Working Group. Here, they continually provide up-to-date information on the foods that are the most heavily contaminated with pesticides and other toxicants. That way, you can make educated choices when buying produce and other foods and help your budget stretch a little further.

In addition to eating only organic foods, the importance of paying attention to the overall health of your gastrointestinal system cannot be understated! You gut is highly innervated and provides a significant supply of critical hormones and neurotransmitters that can make or break your journey to optimum health. You can support your gastrointestinal tract by limiting processed foods, eating naturally fermented foods such as sauerkraut or kefir on a regular basis, take a high-quality probiotic supplement, and eliminating gluten and other gliadin molecules from your diet. For more information, please see Chapter 18.

## 6. Preventing Disease with Lifestyle Changes!

There are simple steps that can be taken to assist in an ongoing program of detox and recovery from heavy metal poisoning. Following are some simple tools and supplements that have been found to be especially useful in supporting your detox endeavors. Please see Chapter 19 for more information.

- Regularly scheduled testing for heavy metals
- Far infrared saunas
- Eating fermented foods/gut health
- Regular exercise

# CHAPTER 13

# Get Tested!

There are various routes that can be used for an accurate analysis of your body burden for heavy metals, the most important include:

- Whole blood, red blood cell and serum minerals
- Urine toxic and essential minerals
- Creatinine clearance
- Hair minerals
- Fecal metals

## Whole Blood, Red Blood Cell and Serum Minerals

Blood testing for heavy metals exposure is the most common methods used in a conventional doctor's office. However, heavy metal testing in blood can only provide information about short-term, high exposures, whereas low-level exposures that occur over a long period of time are far more common. Therefore, analysis of whole blood should primarily be used to assess recent or ongoing exposure to hazardous elements and only to assess acute exposures and to check for appropriate levels of essential minerals. Acute lead and mercury exposure is primarily diagnosed through detection in whole blood. Generally, seven milliliters of whole blood are required to test for heavy metals.

Analysis of red blood cells is used to determine the status of essential minerals that might be affected by heavy metal toxicity and are known to serve important cellular functions. Examples include magnesium, copper, and zinc. Red blood cell analysis can also be used to identify recent exposure to heavy metals that preferentially accumulate there, such as arsenic, cadmium, lead, methylmercury and thallium. Generally, four milliliters of packed red blood cells are required to test for essential minerals in red blood cells.

Analysis of serum elements measures the contents of the blood outside of the red blood cells and clotting factors that make up whole blood. This is useful for measuring electrolytes and extracellular fluids.

(Please see table 3 for specific mineral information for each of these blood components.)

## Urine Toxic and Essential Minerals

The production of urine is one of the primary mechanisms the body has to dispose of waste products that are either made through normal biological pathways or consumed unintentionally from the environment. Therefore, evaluation of urine minerals can give you an idea of the potentially toxic compounds that your body is trying to eliminate. Urine analysis can also be useful to monitor treatments that are being used to help you eliminate the load of heavy metals that you are currently experiencing.

Heavy metal analysis in the urine is usually completed following a "challenge" with a chelating agent. A commonly used chelator is dimercaptosuccinic acid (DMSA), which has also been approved by the U.S. FDA for the treatment of lead poisoning. Once administered, DMSA binds to the heavy metals in the body and is eliminated in the urine, which can then be collected and analyzed. Because DMSA does not bind to other essential minerals such as iron, calcium, magnesium and zinc, it is an excellent compound for this purpose. Generally, 50 milliliters of urine are required for analysis.

## Creatinine Clearance

Many heavy metals, including cadmium, lead and mercury are potent toxicants that affect the kidneys. Because the kidneys serve a very important function in the removal of many different toxic compounds from the body, if their function is compromised by heavy metals then a variety of harmful substances may accumulate in the body. The mobilization of toxic compounds, including heavy metals, using pharmaceutical agents may exacerbate the problem by placing additional stress on the kidneys. Therefore, measurements of creatinine clearance are often performed prior to chelation challenges or other testing methods in individual's that may have reduced kidney function. This allows practitioners to determine appropriate dosage of the chelating agent.

Measurements that examine creatinine clearance are widely used for determining how well your kidneys may be functioning. This test is important for determining how well your body will handle the stress associated with "detoxing" or eliminating the metals that are making you sick.

Table 3. Minerals that are effectively measured in blood (adapted with permission from Doctor's Data, Inc. 2015).

| | Essential MacroMinerals | Essential MicroMinerals | Toxic Heavy Metals |
|---|---|---|---|
| **Comprehensive Blood Minerals** | Calcium Magnesium Sodium Potassium Phosphorus | Copper Zinc Manganese Selenium Molybdenum Iron Cobalt Lithium Chromium | Arsenic Cadmium Lead Mercury Nickel Platinum Thallium Tungsten Uranium Barium Strontium Platinum |
| **Whole Blood Minerals** | Calcium Magnesium | Copper Zinc Manganese Selenium Molybdenum Lithium | Arsenic Cadmium Lead Mercury Nickel Platinum Thallium Tungsten Uranium Barium Strontium |

| **Serum Minerals** | Calcium | Iron | |
| --- | --- | --- | --- |
| | Magnesium | | |
| | Sodium | | |
| | Potassium | | |
| | Phosphorus | | |
| **Red Blood Cell Minerals** | Calcium | Copper | Arsenic |
| | Magnesium | Zinc | Cadmium |
| | Potassium | Manganese | Lead |
| | Phosphorus | Selenium | Mercury |
| | | Molybdenum | Tungsten |
| | | Iron | Vanadium |
| | | Chromium | Boron |

# Hair Elements

In addition to blood analysis, measuring the elements present in the hair is a useful tool for measuring recent and ongoing exposure to heavy metals, especially methylmercury and arsenic. Measuring toxic heavy metal levels in hair samples is an ideal way for checking current exposure levels to toxic metals and allows practitioners to diagnose heavy metal–related disorders earlier than otherwise possible. According to the U.S. EPA (Jenkins 1979):

> … if hair and nail samples are collected, cleaned, and analyzed properly with the best analytical methods under controlled conditions by experienced personnel, the data are valid.

Testing hair samples for heavy metal toxicity is most useful, clinically, to determine if heavy metals are contributing to a disease state. In most other body samples, including blood, urine and fecal matter, the body has tightly regulated mechanisms for overcoming the effects of any type of toxic exposure. Hair samples, however, are not living tissues and are therefore unaffected by these regulatory mechanisms within the body. As a consequence, the heavy metal content in hair samples is often times predictive of an individual's likelihood for developing physical abnormalities in the future.

Hair testing is also useful to determine if deficiencies in any of the essential minerals is present and may also be causing adverse health effects. Testing generally requires 1 gram of clean hair, taken from an area as close to the scalp as possible.

At times, various hair treatments can affect the results of hair measurements and cause a misreading of high or low levels for certain minerals. Table 6 below includes various shampoos that contain high levels of zinc or selenium, which may interfere with normal hair analysis.

Table 4. Zinc- and selenium-containing shampoos (adapted with permission from Genova/Metametrix Clinical Laboratory (2015))

| Zinc-containing shampoo | Selenium-containing shampoo |
| --- | --- |
| • Head & Shoulders® | • Selsum Blue® |
| • Zincon® | • Head & Shoulders Intensive Tx® |
| • Dandrex® | • Selenium sulfide 1% |
| • Subulon | • Selseb |
| • DHS zinc | • Selsun 2.5% |
| • ZNP bar | • Exsel 2.5% |
| • Theraplex Z | • Selenium sulfide 2.5% |

# Fecal Metals

Measuring the heavy metal content of fecal matter will provide a good indication of an individual's exposure through the diet. As such, heavy metal testing in fecal matter will tell you whether or not you are currently being exposed to a heavy metal in "real-time." Also, for many metals fecal excretion is the primary route of elimination from the body; therefore, fecal metal content can indirectly provide information about the overall body burden of heavy metals.

Measuring the heavy metal content in the feces can be a good indicator of how well the body's natural detoxification system is working. This is in contrast to the use of chelating agents that may be administered to bind with heavy metals—which are then excreted in the urine. Consequently, fecal heavy metal analysis might be especially useful to monitor infants or individuals who have inadequate kidney function.

Table 5. Consequences of low blood levels of essential minerals (adapted with permission from Genova/ Metametrix Clinical Laboratory (2015))

| | Symptoms/Disease | Treatment Options |
|---|---|---|
| **Calcium** | • High blood pressure<br>• Oxidative stress | • Magnesium<br>• Omega –3 FA's<br>• Antioxidants |
| **Magnesium** | • Muscle cramping<br>• Depression<br>• High blood pressure<br>• Diabetes | • Supplement |
| **Potassium** | • High blood pressure<br>• Stroke<br>• Kidney stones<br>• Osteoporosis | • Supplement |
| **Iron** | • Fatigue<br>• Cognitive impairments | • Vitamin C<br>• Increase red meats |
| **Zinc** | • Slowed growth<br>• Poor immune function<br>• Hair loss<br>• Diarrhea | • Supplement |
| **Copper** | • Anemia<br>• Diabetic tendencies | • Supplement |
| **Manganese** | • Oxidative stress | • Supplement |
| **Selenium** | • Poor immunity<br>• Decreased fertility<br>• Decreased thyroid function | • Supplement |
| **Molybdenum** | • Sulfite intolerance<br>• Copper Toxicity | • Supplement |
| **Chromium** | • Poorly regulated blood sugar | • Supplement |
| **Cobalt** | • Pernicious Anemia | • Vitamin B12 supplements |
| **Boron** | • Steroid hormone imbalances<br>• Poor bone health<br>• Prostate Cancer | • Supplement |
| **Lithium** | • Psychosis<br>• Depression<br>• Violence<br>• Learning Disabilities | • Supplement |
| **Vanadium** | • Diabetic tendencies | • Supplement |
| **Strontium** | • Osteoporosis | • Supplement |

Table 6. Consequences of high blood levels of essential minerals (adapted with permission from Genova/Metametrix Clinical Laboratory (2015))

|  | Symptoms/Disease | Treatment Options |
|---|---|---|
| **Calcium** | • High blood pressure<br>• Oxidative stress | • Magnesium<br>• Omega -3 FA's<br>• Antioxidants |
| **Iron** | • Vomiting<br>• Bloody diarrhea<br>• Shock<br>• Abdominal Pain | • Decrease iron<br>• Phlebotomy (blood removal) |
| **Zinc** | • Cancer<br>• High Blood Pressure | • Avoid Supplemental zinc |
| **Copper** | • Nausea<br>• Vomiting<br>• Neurodegeneration<br>• Heart Disease | • Zinc Supplementation<br>• Reduce exposure to copper cookware, pipes, and copper-containing medications |
| **Manganese** | • Neurotoxicity | • Decrease intake<br>• EDTA chelation therapy |
| **Selenium** | • Garlic odor on breath<br>• Brittle fingernails<br>• Neurological problems<br>• Swelling | • $B_{12}$ Supplementation |
| **Chromium** | • Dermatitis | • Balance gut microflora |
| **Nickel** | • Cancer<br>• Dermatitis<br>• Asthma<br>• Sinusitis | • Reduce stainless steel cookware<br>• Remove nickel jewelry |
| **Lithium** | • Neurological impairments<br>• Thyroid suppression<br>• Hair loss | • Reduce exposure |
| **Vanadium** | • Respiratory Disorders<br>• Neurological impairment | • Reduce exposure |

If your doctor determines that you have high levels of heavy metals in your system, chelation therapy may be recommended to assist your body in the difficult process of removing them. The following table lists some of the more common chelation agents that may be recommended.

Table 7. Common chelating agents used for removal of toxic heavy metals (adapted with permission from Genova/Metametrix Clinical Laboratory (2015))

| Chelating Agent | Arsenic | Lead | Mercury | Copper | Aluminum | Iron | Cadmium |
|---|---|---|---|---|---|---|---|
| DMPS | ◆ | ◆ | ◆ | | | | |
| DMSA | ◆ | ◆ | ◆ | ◆ | | | |
| BAL | ◆ | ◆ | ◆ | ◆ | | | |
| DPA | ◆ | ◆ | ◆ | ◆ | | | |
| DFO | | | | | ◆ | ◆ | |
| CaNa$_2$-EDTA | ◆ | ◆ | ◆ | | ◆ | | ◆ |

DMPS: 2,3-Dimercapto-1-propane sulfonic acid

DMSA: Meso-2,3-dimercaptosuccinic acid or succimer

BAL: Dimercaprol (British anti-Lewisite)

DPA: D-Penicillamine (Cuprimine, Depen)

DFO: Desferoxamine

CaNa$_2$-EDTA: Calcium disodium ethylenediaminetetraacetic acid

# Chapter 13 References

Doctor's Data Inc. 2015. Toxic and essential elements.

Metametrix Clinical Laboratory. 2015. Elements interpretive guide: blood, hair and urine.

Jenkins, D. 1979. Toxic trace metals in mammalian hair and nails. edited by U.S. Environmental Protection Agency.

# CHAPTER 14

# Get Treated!

## Important Considerations

The concepts outlined in this book rely on the philosophy of functional medicine, which dictates that before we can treat a disease, we have to understand the underlying issues causing the problem. With that in mind, it is important to understand that heavy metal toxicity does not occur in a vacuum. We are all being exposed to many different kinds of environmental toxicants that may be contributing to our health problems. I hope I have made the case in this book for the key role of heavy metals in destroying our health, but for some people there may also be other factors that must be addressed before moving forward with the treatments I suggest in the following pages. For example, mutations in a gene known as methylenetetrahydrofolate reductase (or MTHFR for short) are increasingly being linked to a long laundry list of adverse health conditions ranging from

### Folate and the MTHFR Gene

- The MTHFR gene encodes for the synthesis of an enzyme critical for folate homeostasis
- Mutations in the MTHFR gene are associated with a long list of health problems
- Essential for preventing birth defects during pregnancy
- Important for blood maintenance and prevention of anemia
- Helps to maintain gastrointestinal health
- Important for maintaining good mental health and preventing depression
- Prevents terminal illnesses such as colorectal cancer
- Researchers are continually learning more about the importance of folate for good health

Down's syndrome to miscarriage to depression. This gene encodes for the production of an enzyme protein by the same name that is important for maintaining the homeostasis of folate in the body. Folate is an extremely important molecule in the body for metabolism and promoting healthy cellular growth among other things. If you think you or someone you love may have a mutated MTHFR gene you need to consider that you may experience difficulty in the detox process. Please don't be discouraged! There are additional tests and protocols that may benefit you, including "nutrigenomic" testing that will help identify treatment considerations unique to your specific genetic situation. Additional information can be found in the resource section at the end of this book.

In addition to specific genetic mutations, such as in the MTHFR gene, recent cutting-edge research suggests that some people may be extremely sensitive to multiple environmental toxicants and have a reduced capacity to "detox." Researchers have this to say regarding the issue if you are considering chelation therapy (Flora and Pachauri 2010):

> Chelating agents can affect metal toxicity by mobilizing the toxic metal mainly into urine. A chelating agent forming a stable complex with a toxic metal may shield biological targets from the metal ion, thereby reducing the local toxicity … However, sometimes a chelator may expose the metal to the biological environment and thus increase the toxicity of the metal.

If this happens to you, it is possible that you are a "poor de-toxer," which requires that you pay special attention not to overburden your system. So, if you believe this describes your circumstances, in addition to the heavy metals test, I highly recommend that you undergo an additional series of tests to examine whether or not you are able to tolerate chemicals.

Chemical tolerance is essentially an innate ability to "detox" environmental toxicants and dietary proteins without stimulating an immune response. In particular, if you find that you have an intolerance to strong smells, find it difficult to tolerate routine exposures such as perfumes, detergents, or nickel-containing jewelry; or have regular skin outbreaks and multiple sensitivities it is possible that you have lost your chemical tolerance and must proceed with caution (Kharrazian 2014).

In addition to genetic deficiencies that interfere with your natural ability to detox after a heavy metal or other environmental insult to your body, there are nutritional aspects that can cause similar symptoms and may lead to disease. In particular, there are essential amino acids that your body uses as precursors for the monoamines, serotonin and dopamine, which are critical for the proper functioning of almost every body system. Other essential components of the diet provide precursors for the proper functioning of glutathione and methylation of DNA (a process called epigenetics). Imbalances in one or more of these precursors can lead to catastrophic nutritional deficiencies that may ultimately cause the severe symptoms associated with cancer, Parkinson's disease, depression, autism and many others. Therefore, replenishing the body's supply of these precursors will allow your body to sufficiently produce these "all-important" neurotransmitters and for many people, symptoms can disappear if a competent physician treats your symptoms adequately.

There are several steps that can be taken prior to beginning chelation therapy if you believe you might suffer from a chemical intolerance or nutritional imbalance. First, it is of utmost importance that you find a competent health care provider that specializes in functional medicine and understands the complexities associated with these issues. There are a number of tests that can be done prior to starting chelation therapy that are available through various labs, which can show if your chemical immune tolerance has been lost. If there are positive markers, then it is highly recommended to work on detoxification and building up the immune system before chelation therapy is attempted. Other testing evaluates the integrity of the blood-brain barrier. If testing is positive, then there are concerns of inflammation and serious nutritional changes must be considered first. The next test recommended is one that tests for: "leaky gut syndrome." This can be managed and helped with dietary, nutrition, and lifestyle changes.

# Chelation Therapy

*Background and Description*

Chelation therapy is a method used to "bind" toxic heavy metals within the body so they can be efficiently eliminated through the urinary or fecal waste. In addition, chelation therapy has been shown to help reverse atherosclerosis, prevent heart attacks and strokes (Lamas et al. 2013), and is considered by some to be a safe alternative to bypass surgery and angioplasty (Periasamy et al. 2014).

Because chelation therapy helps remove the body's load of toxic heavy metals and the free-radicals they generate, it can also help reduce systemic inflammation and decrease the amount of oxidative stress that you may be experiencing (Roussel et al. 2009). Decreasing systemic inflammation, in turn, will reduce your risk and symptoms due to degenerative diseases such as arthritis and autoimmune diseases. Chelation therapy can be administered by intravenous (I.V.) infusions or taken orally. Ethylenediaminetetraacetic acid (EDTA) is the most commonly used chelating agent, but it is only approved by the U.S. food and drug administration to treat lead and other heavy metal toxicity. However, there are a growing number of physicians who recommend chelation therapy for cardiovascular and other diseases as well.

Physicians that have been specifically trained in I.V. chelation therapy generally perform the treatment on an outpatient basis. Most doctors recommend twenty to thirty treatments over the course of several weeks. Generally, a very specific supplementation regimen of vitamins and minerals are taken along with the chelation therapy in order to fully optimize the results.

Oral chelation therapy is a viable option for non-emergency removal of heavy metal burdens in the body. Because only a very small percentage of oral EDTA is actually absorbed into the body, the results from oral chelation therapy are generally less dramatic and require longer periods of treatment. However, there are several advantages to oral chelation therapy, including convenience and low cost as well as continuous long-term maintenance of health.

*Chelation Therapy for Heavy Metal Disorders*

The treatment of heavy metal disorders is the most common use of chelation therapy. This includes genetic diseases such thalassemia (which results in iron overload) and Wilson's disease (which results in copper overload), along with the accumulation of other toxic heavy metals in the body.

Chelation therapy is generally designed to "systemically" remove the toxic heavy metals from the entire body and has shown promise for the treatment of other conditions described more below. There are various types of chelating agents that may be prescribed, depending on an individual's specific heavy metal burden (see Table 7 for more information).

*Chelation Therapy and the Brain*

Many of the most debilitating effects of heavy metal poisoning are neurological in nature. Disorders range from deficits in learning, memory and movement to severe and even fatal neurological diseases. In addition to acute toxic effects, many heavy metals disrupt the balance of other essential minerals, such as zinc, copper and iron. It has been proposed that the combination of these two events may contribute to certain degenerative diseases such as Alzheimer's disease (Budimir 2011). This idea is supported by the observation that unusually high levels of iron (Loef and Walach 2012) and imbalances in the levels of zinc and copper (Loef, von Stillfried, and Walach 2012) are commonly found in the brain of people who have died from Alzheimer's disease. All three of these metals (copper, iron and zinc) are commonly associated with the protein "plaques" that often leads to a diagnosis of Alzheimer's disease. Therefore, removal of heavy metals from the body through chelation therapy may assist in the "redistribution" and proper balance of other essential minerals and, in turn, improve the outlook for patients with Alzheimer's and other neurological diseases.

*Chelation Therapy and the Heart*

One of the most important studies relating to chelation therapy was recently published in the Journal of the American Medical

Association. Referred to as "TACT" (for **T**rial to **A**ssess **C**helation **T**herapy), this was the first randomized, multi-center, long-term and double blind (all the hallmarks of a top-notch study design) study on the benefits of chelation therapy (ClinicalTrials.gov 2013). The study was sponsored by the Mt. Sinai Medical Center in Miami and included collaborators from the National Heart, Blood and Lung Institute as well as the National Center for Complementary and Alternative Medicine. According to the National Institute of Health, the trial included 1,708 patients who had been enrolled from September 2003 through October 2011. Participants were recruited from 134 sites within the United States and Canada. The study only included patients who previously had experienced a heart attack and ultimately demonstrated that the patients receiving chelation therapy had fewer cardiovascular disease complications than those who received placebo infusions. Needless to say, TACT was designed to evaluate the impact of chelation therapy on coronary artery disease and included four treatment categories (also summarized in table 8): 1) patients who received EDTA chelation therapy, 2) patients who received chelation therapy but with a placebo instead of EDTA, 3) patients who received EDTA or placebo chelation therapy plus a high dose vitamin supplement and 4) patients who received EDTA or placebo chelation therapy plus a high dose vitamin placebo. The results from TACT have caused a significant amount of passionate discussion among health care providers in both the conventional and alternative worlds of medicine.

There are many interesting insights that can be illustrated simply by looking at the basic outcomes of the study. For example, even the enrollment data shows interesting trends. One of the criticisms of this study has been that it is an unfeasible treatment regime that is too rigorous. In other words, it doesn't matter if it is an effective treatment if people won't follow through with it. However, a look at the actual data tells a different story. According to publically available information (ClinicalTrials.gov, 2013), the highest dropout numbers were actually in the group of people who were receiving the placebo treatment. This group was almost twice the number of individuals who were receiving the chelation therapy and still chose to leave the study. We cannot interview these individuals, so we do not know for certain what their reasons for dropping out might have been, but it is worth speculating that the group receiving EDTA were experiencing noticeable benefits that the placebo group did not experience.

> "But early in my career, I became discouraged by the severe limitations of conventional medicine. Instead of curing our patients, we could only offer them the equivalent of extended "life support.""
>
> –Dr. Roy Heilbron (Cardiologist)
> (TACT Researcher & Author of *Healing Heart Disease With Chelation Therapy*)

It is of significance to note that the primary endpoint of the trial was significantly lowered in the EDTA chelated group. The studied endpoint was an overall measurement of adverse cardiac events, including: death, myocardial infarction, coronary revascularization, and hospitalization for angina. The most significant benefits were noted in patients with diabetes; the number of adverse cardiac events recorded for diabetic patients undergoing EDTA chelation therapy was 67 compared to 102 events for the placebo group. Significantly, a second study focusing specifically on the benefits of chelation therapy in diabetics is being organized and is expected to begin enrollment in late 2015 or early 2016!

In addition to the significant improvement in the number of adverse cardiac events observed among patients undergoing chelation therapy, an important aspect of TACT was the establishment of chelation therapy as a safe medical treatment. In fact, according to publically available information about the study, patients receiving chelation therapy did not suffer more from complications of the GI tract, immune system, kidneys or nutritional deficiencies than patients receiving the placebo treatments (ClinicalTrials.gov, 2013).

# Benefits of Chelation

While the benefits of chelation therapy are not highly publicized, there is a huge body of peer-reviewed literature (over 500 publications) supporting the positive health benefits to people who use it. The following is a list of the most notable effects that have been proven through research on chelation therapy (Oradix 2015):

- Antiaging: There are a lot of cellular processes that contribute to the antiaging effects attributed to chelation therapy, but overall, the result is a longer life expectancy with increased energy
- Cosmetic changes: Believe it or not, chelation therapy has been shown to improve the luster and strength of hair fibers, strengthen nails; improve skin color, texture and tone; lighten age spots and reduce wrinkles. Overall, the result is a more youthful appearance
- Improves taste, vision and hearing
- Helps to prevent (or even reverse) "hardening of the arteries" or arteriosclerosis: Chelation therapy does this by preventing the oxidative damage caused by heavy metals. In addition, it directly removes calcium and plaque build-up
- Improves the overall cardiovascular system: Chelation therapy has been shown to reduce blood pressure, chest pain, arrhythmias and cholesterol levels
- Reduces the damage caused by electro-magnetic radiation: Electromagnetic radiation is emitted by various sources, including cell phones, cell phone towers, WiFi and microwave ovens. This damage caused by this type of radiation is compounded in the presence of heavy metals
- Antimicrobial activity: EDTA in-and-of-itself has antimicrobial properties. But, in addition to its own activity, EDTA disrupts the "biofilm" that is formed by microbes in the body that serves as a critical component of their defense system. In fact, EDTA has shown better anti-fungal properties than specific antifungal drugs, including nystatin ketoconazole. This means that chelation therapy is highly beneficial in the treatment of candida infections

- Restore the normal distribution of essential minerals: The accumulation of toxic heavy metals interferes with the normal distribution and availability of essential minerals and elements such as zinc, cobalt, chromium etc. Therefore, removal of these toxic metals through chelation therapy allows the body to re-establish normal levels of these important elements
- Rebalance hormones: Similar to the havoc on essential minerals and elements caused by excessive heavy metals in your system, a hormonal imbalance is often seen as well. When essential elements are not properly balanced, "vitamins are useless and enzymes cannot function properly." This, in turn, leads to disruptions in hormonal levels
- Lowers insulin requirements for diabetics
- Improves post-surgery recovery time
- Provides relief from leg muscle cramps
- Reduces allergy symptoms
- Helps to normalize weight
- Reduces anxiety, depression and hyperactivity
- Reduces reliance on pain medication
- Improves kidney function: Chelation therapy helps to dissolve kidney stones and reduces varicose veins
- Improves mental clarity: Chelation therapy improves the microcirculation of the brain, reduces the effects of infections, and reduces the heavy metal burden that directly damages the nervous system (i.e. mercury and lead). In combination, these effects result in a higher mental acuity
- Benefits to the prostate
- Assists in poor circulation, therefore extremities feel "warmer"
- Reduces cancer mortality
- Reduces oxidative damage to cells

## Forms of Chelation Therapy

*Intravenous (IV) Chelation Therapy*

For emergency care of heavy metal toxicity, intravenous chelation therapy will garner the most rapid results. However, treatments can often times be costly and time-consuming. In addition, few insurance policies will cover chelation therapy at this time. As such, IV chelation therapy is the most expensive type, both in terms of finances and time required. Generally, IV chelation requires anywhere from 30-50 sessions over a period of six months. In that time, you will receive 3000 mg of EDTA per session. Each session requires around 3 hours of your time and costs anywhere from $100-$150. Increasingly, practitioners are choosing other methods for chelation therapy because the introduction of EDTA into the system by IV administration can be overwhelming to many patients who are unable to deal with the rapid mobilization of heavy metals. Nonetheless, chelation clinics that administer IV therapy take extra measures, such as giving additional vitamin C, to counteract the difficulties associated with the rapid removal of toxicants such as heavy metals.

In short, many practitioners feel that IV chelation therapy lacks the necessary flexibility required of many patients, while the price is often prohibitively high. However, other methods of chelation therapy may serve the majority of patients well.

*Chelation Suppositories*

Increasingly, chelation suppositories are replacing IV chelation as the preferred method. Benefits include flexibility, lower costs and better absorption of the EDTA during the night. In addition, chelation suppositories are considered by some to be the equivalent to the more traditional IV delivery of EDTA (Ellithorpe et al. 2007). If you choose to take advantage of EDTA in suppository form, it is typically administered every other night. According to chelation researchers (Pelletier):

> Suppositories provide direct access to the systemic circulation, efficiently bypassing portal circulation and liver metabolism via the hemorrhoidal veins.

The use of chelation suppositories is also gaining momentum for the treatment of heavy metal–related diseases. For example, EDTA in suppository form was shown to significantly reduce pain associated pelvic pain syndrome (prostatitis) in combination with tetracycline (an antibiotic) (Ellithorpe et al. in review). It is known that heavy metals may contribute to prostate cancer (Kazantzis 1981); therefore, it is believed that EDTA suppositories are effective in treating prostatitis partially due to the removal of heavy metals within the system.

Chelation suppositories also represent a promising treatment for children that have been exposed to high levels of lead and are at significant risk for mental deficiencies. Suppositories are ideal for treating children because they are highly effective, but do not pose the same potential risks that are associated with IV chelation therapy. In addition, chelation suppositories are "fast-acting" compared to oral chelators—a critical characteristic for agents used to remove lead from children.

As opposed to IV chelation therapy, the use of EDTA suppositories presents the following advantages (Pelletier et al.):

- More opportunities to bind to heavy metals
- The ability to space out the maximum recommended dose of EDTA over one week (instead of two days), which greatly improves its effectiveness
- Improved safety—EDTA suppositories do not cause critical deficiencies in blood serum calcium levels

*Oral Chelation*

Over the long-term, oral chelation can be just as effective as intravenous chelation therapy. However, oral EDTA is poorly absorbed, requiring its use over many years in order to equal the benefits of IV or suppository chelation therapy in the short term. While oral chelators were not included in the highly publicized TACT study, healthcare practitioners have successfully and safely used them for many decades. In fact, oral EDTA therapy has been used since the 1940's to treat lead poisoning. Oral chelation is, in fact, a viable option for treatment of non-emergency heavy metal overload.

# Chapter 14 References

Oradix. 2015. "Get the most out of chelation." Oradix Accessed February 2, 2015. http://oradix.com/pages/24-Benefits-of-Chelation.html.

Budimir, A. 2011. "Metal ions, Alzheimer's disease and chelation therapy." *Acta pharmaceutica* 61 (1):1-14. doi: 10.2478/v10007-011-0006-6.

ClinicalTrials.gov. 2013. "Trial to assess chelation therapy (TACT)." Accessed November 19, 2014. http://clinicaltrials.gov/ct2/show/results/NCT00044213?sect=X430156 - othr.

Ellithorpe, R., L. Clapp, T. Jimenez, B. Jacques, R. Settineri, and G.L. Nicolson. in review. "Anti-microbial plus CaNa2EDTA chelation suppository therapy for chronic prostatitis/pelvic pain syndrome with or without prostatic hyperplasia: preliminary study." *World Journal of Urology*.

Ellithorpe, R., P. Mazur, G. Gum, G. Button, J. Le, E.H. Pfadenhauer, R.A. Settineri, and G. Nicolson. 2007. "Comparison of the absorption, brain and prostate distribution, and elimination of CaNa2 EDTA of rectal chelation suppositories to intravenous administration." *The Journal of the American Nutraceutical Association* 10 (2):5-12.

Flora, S. J., and V. Pachauri. 2010. "Chelation in metal intoxication." *International journal of environmental research and public health* 7 (7):2745-88. doi: 10.3390/ijerph7072745.

Kazantzis, G. 1981. "Role of cobalt, iron, lead, manganese, mercury, platinum, selenium, and titanium in carcinogenesis." *Environmental health perspectives* 40:143-61.

Kharrazian, D. 2014. "Title." *drknews.com*, December 10, 2014. http://drknews.com/chelation-autoimmunity/.

Lamas, G. A., C. Goertz, R. Boineau, D. B. Mark, T. Rozema, R. L. Nahin, L. Lindblad, E. F. Lewis, J. Drisko, and K. L. Lee. 2013. "Effect of disodium EDTA chelation regimen on cardiovascular events in patients with previous myocardial infarction: the TACT randomized trial." *JAMA: the journal of the American Medical Association* 309 (12):1241-50. doi: 10.1001/jama.2013.2107.

Loef, M., N. von Stillfried, and H. Walach. 2012. "Zinc diet and Alzheimer's disease: a systematic review." *Nutritional neuroscience* 15 (5):2-12. doi: 10.1179/1476830512Y.0000000010.

Loef, M., and H. Walach. 2012. "Copper and iron in Alzheimer's disease: a systematic review and its dietary implications." *The British journal of nutrition* 107 (1):7-19. doi: 10.1017/S000711451100376X.

Pelletier, M., J. Lavalle, R. Ellithorpe, M. Schmidt, R. Pelton, and R. Settineri. "Effects of CaNa2EDTA (Detoxamin®) suppositories on excretion of heavy metals." Cincinnati, OH.

Periasamy, V. S., J. Athinarayanan, A. M. Al-Hadi, F. A. Juhaimi, and A. A. Alshatwi. 2014. "Effects of Titanium Dioxide Nanoparticles Isolated from Confectionery Products on the Metabolic Stress Pathway in Human Lung Fibroblast Cells." *Archives of environmental contamination and toxicology.* doi: 10.1007/s00244-014-0109-4.

Roussel, A. M., I. Hininger-Favier, R. S. Waters, M. Osman, K. Fernholz, and R. A. Anderson. 2009. "EDTA chelation therapy, without added vitamin C, decreases oxidative DNA damage and lipid peroxidation." *Alternative medicine review: a journal of clinical therapeutic* 14 (1):56-61.

# CHAPTER 15

# Remove and Avoid Sources of Exposure

Fish are not the only source for heavy metals encountered in our everyday lives. This chapter will outline additional places where exposure may take place as well as introduce you to metals that are considered rare, but may still be very toxic as well as help you find a balance for essential metals. Take for example, the following tables of common household items:

Table 10. Metals in commonly used cookware (mg/L).

|  | Aluminum | Chrome | Cobalt | Nickel | Leaching? |
|---|---|---|---|---|---|
| **Non-Stick Anodized Aluminum** | 7.10 |  |  |  | Yes |
| **Ceramic Non-Stick Aluminum Skillet** | 1.40 |  |  | 0.95 | Yes |
| **Seasoned Cast Iron Skillet** |  | 2.08 |  | 2,817.00 | Yes |
| **Anodized Aluminum** |  |  | 3.28 |  | Yes |

Table 11. Metals commonly found in beauty and hygiene products (adapted with permission from Genova/Metametrix Clinical Laboratory (2015)).

| Products with Heavy Metals | Name on the Label | Health Concerns |
|---|---|---|
| • Lip products<br>• Eyeliner<br>• Foundation<br>• Eye shadow<br>• Concealer<br>• Eye drops<br>• Whitening toothpaste<br>• Nail color<br>• Sunscreen<br>• Blush<br>• Moisturizer | • Lead acetate<br>• Thimerosal<br>• Sodium hexametaphosphate<br>• Chromium<br>• Hydrogenated cotton seed oil | • Cancer<br>• Reproductive toxicity<br>• Allergies<br>• Bioaccumulation<br>• Developmental toxicity<br>• Organ system toxicity<br>• Immunotoxicity |

## Potentially Toxic and Rare Earth Metals

In addition to the toxic heavy metals that are addressed in this book, there are other metals that are less common or even rare earth metals that may cause toxic effects. The following tables address some of these elements.

Table 12. Rare metals and potentially toxic metals used in the medical industry (adapted with permission from Genova/Metametrix Clinical Laboratory (2015))

| Metal | Medical Source | Symptoms | Possible Treatments |
|---|---|---|---|
| **Antimony** | Some anti-helminthic drugs | Fatigue, headaches, metallic taste, abdominal pain, anemia, low back pain | Avoidance, BAL, DMSA, glutathione, or N-acetylcysteine |
| **Barium** | X-ray contrast media, Enema salts | Gastrointestinal complaints, muscle weakness, facial numbness, low blood pressure | Oral sodium sulfate |

| | | | |
|---|---|---|---|
| **Bismuth** | OTC medications, X-ray contrast media | Nausea, vomiting, diarrhea | BAL or penicillamine for chelation |
| **Cerium** | Dental compositions | Itching, sensitivity to heat, skin lesions | Avoidance and treatment of symptoms |
| **Europium** | Genetic disease testing | Skin and lung irritation | Avoidance and treat symptoms |
| **Indium** | Diagnostic nuclear medicine | Lung inflammation, reproductive effects | Avoidance and treat symptoms |
| **Niobium** | Joint replacements, dental implants | Possible lung irritation, skin sensitization | Avoidance and treat symptoms |
| **Palladium** | Dental alloys | Possible lung inflammation, skin sensitization, allergic reaction | Avoidance and treat symptoms |
| **Platinum** | Surgical tools, dental restorations, chemotherapy drugs, silicone breast implants | Contact dermatitis, respiratory symptoms | Avoidance and treat symptoms |
| **Tantalum** | Dental and surgical implants | Skin and eye irritation, lung irritation, lung disease | Avoidance and treat symptoms |
| **Tin** | Dental amalgams | Neurotoxicity; eye, skin and GI irritation, anemia, muscle weakness, testicular degeneration | Avoidance, Selenium supplementation |
| **Tungsten** | X-ray targets | Pulmonary fibrosis, lung cancer, cognitive deficits; reproductive, neurological and developmental effects | Avoidance and treat symptoms |
| **Zirconium** | Surgical appliances, poison ivy lotion | Skin and pulmonic granulomas | Avoidance |

Table 13. Rare metals and potentially toxic metals (adapted with permission from Genova/Metametrix Clinical Laboratory (2015))

| Potential Food contaminant | Potential Contaminant of Cosmetics | Commonly found in Household Items | Commonly used in Jewelry Manufacturing |
|---|---|---|---|
| Antimony | Antimony | Antimony | Niobium |
| Barium | Bismuth | Cerium | Palladium |
| Cerium | Tin | Holmium | Platinum |
| Palladium | | Niobium | Zirconium |
| Rubidium | | Palladium | |
| Tellurium | | Platinum | |
| Tin | | Rubidium | |
| | | Tellurium | |
| | | Thorium | |
| | | Tin | |
| | | Tungsten | |
| | | Zirconium | |

Table 14. Rare metals and potentially toxic metals (adapted with permission from Genova/Metametrix Clinical Laboratory (2015))

| Metal | Sources | Symptoms | Treatment |
|---|---|---|---|
| **Cesium** | Rocks, soil and dust, atomic clocks, fly ash | GI distress, low blood pressure, numbness, ventricular tachycardia, cardiac arrest in severe cases | Avoidance and treat symptoms |
| **Samarium** | Production of synthetic products, cobalt alloys, industrial sources | Skin and eye irritation, GI symptoms, CNS symptoms, cardiac dysfunction | Avoidance and treat symptoms |
| **Terbium** | Lasers, semiconductor devices, phosphors in color television tubes | Eye and skin irritant, digestive tract irritation, respiratory tract irritation | Avoidance and treat symptoms |
| **Thorium** | Naturally occurs in rocks, soil, water, plants and animals; gas mantles for lanterns, tungsten wire coating, camera lenses, welding rods, light bulb filaments, Nuclear energy fuel | Lung disease; increased lung, prostate, bone, and blood cancers; skin irritation | Avoidance and treat symptoms |
| **Thulium** | Industrial sources, microwaves, lasers | Irritation to respiratory tract; damage to GI tract, skin, eyes, or lung; asthma | Avoidance and treat symptoms |
| **Uranium** | Widespread use in military and industry as well as nuclear power | Renal damage, lung cancer | Avoidance, IV sodium bicarbonate inositol hexaphosphate |

# Metal Reference Information

The following is information on many common minerals. Some of them are essential to your good health and others should be avoided completely.

*Aluminum*    Al

- Aluminum is found in beverages that are sold in aluminum cans such as soda pop and beer as well as in food cooked in aluminum cookware. Aluminum is also found in antacids, anti-perspirants, baking powder, many drying agents, processed cheeses and bleached flour. Frequently, municipal water is treated with aluminum and fluoridation of the water increases leaching from aluminum cookware.
- Aluminum is a non-essential, toxic metal.
- Mild and early-onset of symptoms caused by aluminum exposure include excess gas, headaches, digestive upset, dry skin and mucous membranes, susceptibility to colds and heartburn. Early symptoms of aluminum toxicity include: flatulence, headaches, colic, dryness of skin and mucous membranes, tendency for colds, burning pain in head relieved by food, heartburn and an aversion to meat.
- Severe and late-onset of symptoms caused by aluminum exposure include muscle paralysis, memory loss and mental confusion.

*Arsenic*   As

- Arsenic is found in several forms, including organic arsenic, referred to as arsenate, and inorganic arsenite. Arsenate is found in many foods, whereas arsenite is typically found in pesticides, paint, cosmetics, color pigments, rodenticides, fungicides, wood preservatives and commercial chicken feed. Arsenite can also be found in beer, table salt and water.
- Generally, arsenic is considered to be a non-essential metalloid. However, some laboratories have suggested that arsenic is an essential element in very small quantities.
- Exposure to arsenic interferes with the metabolism of folic acid and the sulfhydryl enzymes that are crucial for innate detoxification. Arsenic is also known to be an effective enzyme inhibitor.
- Arsenic is known to accumulate in the hair.

## Boron   B

- Boron is found in leafy vegetables as well as fruits and nuts. Other sources typically include nuts and legumes as well as alcoholic beverages including wine, cider and beer.
- Boron has several functions in the body. It is important in the production of estrogen and testosterone and is therefore thought to be important in the prevention of osteoporosis and post-menopausal symptoms. Similarly, if you are deficient in boron, you may suffer from symptoms of osteoporosis, hot flashes and vaginal dryness.
- In general, boron is considered a relatively safe element. However, if excessive amounts are consumed, boron may affect calcium metabolism.

## Cadmium    Cd

- Exposure to cadmium can often result from eating food grown on soil contaminated by sewage sludge, cadmium-based fertilizers and irrigation run-off. In addition, cadmium accumulates in the meat of large ocean fish and is often found in processed foods and meat. Cigarettes typically contain high concentrations of cadmium as well. Other sources may include soldered cans, car exhaust, paint and air pollution.
- Cadmium is considered to be a toxic, non-essential heavy metal.
- It is common for newborns to have significant stores of cadmium that have been passed from mother to child during the gestational period.
- Cadmium exposure can have an adverse impact on nearly every major system in the body, including: the nervous, cardiovascular, skeletal, digestive, reproductive, endocrine and excretory systems.

## Calcium    Ca

- Calcium can be found in various sources of food, including seafood (sardines, caviar and smelt), eggs, nuts, seeds and dairy products. Other sources include various vegetables such as kale, mustard and turnip greens, and collards. Brewer's yeast, torula yeast, molasses and kelp can also provide calcium when consumed in the diet.
- The majority of the calcium found in your body is used in the formation of bones. However, calcium is also known to be a key player in other important pathways in the body:

  ❖ Calcium is important for regulating cell membranes which can affect muscle contractions and nerve impulses
  ❖ Calcium is also important in regulating body fluids—affecting the ability of the blood to clot as well as pH (acidity and/or alkalinity)
  ❖ Calcium serves a role in cell division
  ❖ Calcium is important in the regulation of insulin

- When an individual is deficient in calcium, symptoms such as enhanced adrenalin responses, irritability, anxiety and nervousness may be apparent. Other typical signs include muscle cramps and spasms, a tendency to bruise, osteoporosis, high blood pressure, tooth decay and insomnia.
- If calcium is consumed in excessive amounts, then symptoms of apathy, depression, fatigue, and social withdrawal may occur. In addition, arthritis, hardening of arteries and kidney stones are common.
- Absorption of calcium is improved in the presence of vitamin D, along with a sufficiently acidic stomach and protein consumption. Magnesium, copper and vitamin C are all important for assisting the body in its utilization of calcium.

*Chromium*     Cr

- Chromium is commonly found in oysters, egg yolk, peanuts, grape juice, American cheese, wheat and wheat germ. Other sources may include calves' liver, molasses, black pepper and brewer's yeast.
- Chromium is especially important in maintenance of optimal blood sugar, which is also important for ideal energy levels. A role for chromium in the regulation of cholesterol has also been described.
- Chromium also plays an important role in other systems within the body, including:

  ❖ Supplying energy for muscular contraction
  ❖ As an essential component of bones and hair
  ❖ As a protective component within the immune system
  ❖ In the metabolism of fat, protein, and carbohydrates

- A deficiency in chromium may result in elevated serum cholesterol levels, atherosclerosis, stunted growth, fatigue, diabetes, and hypoglycemia.
- In contrast, excessive intakes of chromium can cause asthma, allergies and sinusitis. Other possible outcomes include kidney damage, ulcers, calcium deficiency, vomiting and diarrhea.
- For chromium to function properly in the body, it requires adequate levels of magnesium, vitamin B6, zinc, and manganese.

*Cobalt*    Co

- Cobalt is primarily consumed as vitamin B12 that is found in meat. External sources of cobalt (such as through meat consumption) are necessary for your body to synthesize vitamin B12, which serves important roles in blood formation and the proper functioning of the nervous system.
- People who suffer from deficiencies in cobalt are commonly found to have pernicious anemia. Excessive exposures to cobalt may result in cardiomyopathy.

## Copper    Cu

- Copper is found in many common food sources such as seafood, other meats, nuts and seeds, vegetables, and grains. Copper is also frequently found in yeast, gelatin, chocolate and corn oil. Other potential sources of exposure include leaching from copper water pipes, water additives, some prenatal vitamins and copper cookware.
- Certain medications include copper, such as many birth control pills and intrauterine devices.
- Copper is considered an essential element, but can have severe side effects if consumed in excess.
- Vegetarians and individuals under high levels of stress tend to accumulate copper.
- Copper is an essential element that plays an important role in the production of energy and blood formation as well as the female reproductive system.
- Many children are born with excessive levels of copper due to passage from their mother *in utero*.
- Deficiencies in copper may result in the following symptoms:

  ❖ anemia
  ❖ hair loss
  ❖ atherosclerosis
  ❖ impaired collagen formation
  ❖ demyelination
  ❖ edema
  ❖ osteoporosis

- Excessive consumption of copper may result in the following symptoms:

  ❖ acne
  ❖ adrenal insufficiency
  ❖ mood swings
  ❖ allergies
  ❖ multiple sclerosis

- ❖ migraine headaches
- ❖ heart disease
- ❖ pancreatic dysfunction
- ❖ autism
- ❖ tooth decay
- ❖ depression
- ❖ urinary tract infections
- ❖ diabetes
- ❖ vitamin deficiencies

*Iron*　　Fe

- Iron is found in many common food sources, including seafood, other meats, nuts and seeds, vegetables and grains. Other sources may include red wine, molasses, bone meal and yeast.
- Iron is considered to be an essential metal, but can cause adverse effects if consumed in excess amounts.
- The primary roles of iron in the body include: transportation of oxygen through its role in hemoglobin function, the production of cellular energy and as a component of enzymes important for removing free radicals.
- Excessive iron may result in the following symptoms:

  ❖ arthritis
  ❖ high blood pressure
  ❖ cancer
  ❖ liver cirrhosis
  ❖ diabetes
  ❖ schizophrenia

*Lead*  Pb

- Common sources for lead exposure include cigarette smoke, ceramic glazes, lead-soldered food cans, battery manufacturing, leaded-water pipes, pesticide residues, hair dyes, contaminated water and soil as well as lead-based paint.
- Lead is considered to be an extremely toxic, non-essential heavy metal.
- Many children are born with elevated blood lead levels that are passed to them from the mother during the gestational period.
- Dietary deficiencies in calcium, iron or magnesium facilitate the absorption of lead.
- Lead is an extremely toxic metal that has adverse effects on many systems within the body. In particular, the nervous system is extremely sensitive to lead exposure, as are the cardiovascular, digestive and reproductive systems.

## Lithium   Li

- Lithium is a common element found in a variety of foods. It is also found in various other sources such as lubricating grease, batteries, ceramics and glass. Lithium is also commonly used for the treatment of bipolar disorder to decrease the manic symptoms of patients who suffer from manic-depressive episodes.
- It has been suggested that lithium is important in the formation of prostaglandins from essential fatty acids and helps to stabilize serotonin, both of which may contribute to a decline in aggressive activity when proper lithium levels are attained.
- A Lithium deficiency is commonly associated with aggressive tendencies as well as manic states and depression.
- Excessive consumption of lithium may result in fluid imbalances, nausea, tremors, confusion, disorientation, and possibly seizures, coma and/or death.

*Molybdenum*   Mo

- Molybdenum is a common element found in meat, nuts/seeds and legumes. Grains are also a good source of molybdenum. Exposure to molybdenum can also occur through occupational sources such as the production of stainless steel, lubricants and in photographic chemicals.
- Molybdenum is considered an "ultra-trace" mineral, meaning it is only required in extremely small quantities within the body. The body uses molybdenum primarily to assist with proper copper metabolism.
- Molybdenum deficiencies may result in stunted growth, tooth decay, elevated copper levels and male impotence
- An excessive intake of molybdenum may cause severe diarrhea, gout, as well as symptoms of copper deficiency

## Magnesium    Mg

- Magnesium is commonly found in many nuts such as almonds, Brazil nuts and cashews. Additional sources of magnesium include soybeans, parsnips and grains. Chocolate, cocoa and brewer's yeast are also known to contain magnesium.
- Magnesium plays a vital role in the skeletal system, which is where 60 percent of the body's magnesium is stored. Magnesium is also a critical element for muscle contraction, nerve impulse and to balance the activity of calcium in the body.
- Magnesium is known to act as a laxative agent and for glucose and fat metabolism as well as protein synthesis. Magnesium is also an important agent for proper liver function.
- A deficiency in magnesium will often result in anxiety, irritability, fast heart rate, kidney stones, muscle spasms, irregular heartbeat and tissue calcification.
- Excessive intakes of magnesium may result in confusion, lethargy, depression, muscle weakness, diarrhea and fatigue.

## *Manganese*  Mn

- Manganese is commonly found in egg yolk, nuts/seeds (such as sunflower seeds, coconut, pecans, walnuts, chestnuts, almonds, Brazil nuts and hazelnuts), fruits, corn, legumes and grains. Other sources may include kelp, cloves and tea.
- Manganese plays a vital role in the body for energy production, glucose regulation, and bone development. It is also a key element in the synthesis of neurotransmitters, adrenal and thyroid activity as well as in fertility.
- A manganese deficiency may result in the onset of allergies, hypoglycemia, diabetes, dizziness, fatigue and osteoporosis.
- An excessive intake of manganese may cause a loss of appetite, neurological symptoms, schizophrenia and iron deficiency

*Mercury*    Hg

- The most common sources of mercury exposure are dental amalgams, consumption of large ocean fish, drinking water and agriculture products treated with mercurial fungicides. Some medications can result in mercury exposure as well, including some diuretics, mercurochrome, merthiolate and Preparation H.
- Mercury is considered to be a highly toxic, non-essential heavy metal.
- Many children are born with high levels of systemic mercury due to the transfer of maternal mercury load through the placenta to the child *in utero*. Mercury can also be passed from mother to child through breast milk.
- Copper and zinc deficiencies are often associated with high levels of mercury exposure.
- Mercury toxicity primarily targets the nervous, endocrine and metabolic body systems.
- Symptoms that may be associated with mercury exposure may include:

  ❖ birth defects
  ❖ brain damage
  ❖ depression
  ❖ immune system dysfunction
  ❖ kidney damage
  ❖ memory loss
  ❖ numbness and tingling in arms and legs
  ❖ schizophrenia
  ❖ thyroid dysfunction
  ❖ tremors
  ❖ muscle weakness

*Nickel*   Ni

- Common sources for exposure to nickel include cigarette smoke, nickel-plated cookware, and the manufacturing of steel, batteries and electrical parts. Common food sources include commercial peanut butter, hydrogenated vegetable oils, unrefined grains, vegetarian products, margarine and certain sea products such as kelp.
- Nickel tends to accumulate in the kidneys.
- There is disagreement as to whether or not nickel is an essential element at low concentrations. Suggested functions include a role in hormone, lipid and membrane metabolism.
- Common conditions associated with nickel toxicity include:

  ❖ cancer
  ❖ low blood pressure
  ❖ heart disease
  ❖ muscle tremors
  ❖ nausea and vomiting
  ❖ kidney dysfunction

*Phosphorus*    P

- Phosphorus is commonly found in a variety of seafood, including: anchovies, bass, bluefish, carp, caviar, eel, halibut, herring, mackerel, pike, salmon, sardines, scallops, shad, smelt, trout and tuna. Phosphorus is also commonly found in other meat sources as well as many nuts and seeds. Legumes, grains, chocolate, kelp, cheese, yeast and bone meal are also common sources of phosphorus.
- The vast majority (80-85 percent) of the phosphorus in the body is located in the bones and teeth. Phosphorus is a critical component in energy production, cell membranes as well as the basic genetic material.
- A deficiency in phosphorus is often associated with symptoms of arthritis, tooth decay, fatigue, poor growth, muscle weakness, fragile bones and reproductive problems.
- Excessive ingestion of phosphorus may result in anemia due to iron deficiency, irritability, calcium and magnesium deficiencies, diarrhea and zinc deficiency.

*Potassium*   K

- Sources of potassium include meat and seafood, along with various nuts and seeds. Potassium can also be found in avocados, raisins, prunes, dates and figs. Vegetable sources of potassium include artichokes, beet greens, collard greens, garlic, horseradish, lentils, lima beans, Swiss chard, parsley and potatoes. Potassium can also be found in grains, chocolate, kelp, molasses, mushrooms, salt substitutes and yeast.
- Potassium serves many functions in the body, including effects on the heart rate and blood pressure, maintaining an acid/base balance, adequate digestion, hormone balance and carbohydrate metabolism.
- A deficiency in potassium may result in low blood pressure, constipation, muscle weakness, fatigue, hypoglycemia and water retention.
- Excessive intakes of potassium are generally associated with depression, muscle spasms and diabetes.

## *Selenium*  Se

- Selenium is commonly found in a variety of seafood, including carp, cod, flounder, herring, lobster, mackerel, oysters, pike, salmon, scallops and shrimp. Other meats along with nuts, seeds, grains and brewer's yeast are often good sources of selenium as well.
- Selenium is used within the body to support its antioxidant reserves and to assist with the normal functions of vitamin E. Selenium can be a useful agent in the process of heavy metal detoxification, particularly in the removal of mercury cadmium, silver and arsenic.
- A deficiency in selenium may result in abnormal red blood cells, alcoholic liver, and jaundice in the case of newborns.
- Excessive selenium is often associated with depression, nervousness, gastrointestinal distress, dermatitis, mottled teeth and liver damage.

## Sodium    Na

- Sodium is often found is seafood and other meat sources, such as brains, beef kidney and liver, caviar, clams, eggs, sardines, scallops, shrimp and tuna. Sodium can also be found in several sources of vegetables, including beet greens, celery, olives, peas and Swiss chard. Some dairy products such as butter and cheese, along with common condiments often contain a significant amount of sodium.
- Sodium serves an important function in fluid and blood pressure regulation, maintaining acid–base balance and minimizing the effects of toxic agents by keeping them soluble in body fluids.
- Sodium deficiencies can result in fatigue, lack of appetite, low blood pressure, apathy, bloating, poor protein digestion, depression, dizziness and weakness.
- Excessive sodium intake may be associated with edema, irritability, headaches, nervousness, lowered calcium and magnesium levels, high blood pressure and water retention.

## *Zinc* Zn

- Zinc can commonly be found in beef, herring, lamb, oysters and pork liver. Other sources include sunflower and pumpkin seeds, cheese, wheat germ, bone meal, tea, maple syrup and brewer's yeast.
- Zinc serves an important function in the activation of many enzymes that play a role in growth and development, insulin production and the male reproductive system. Sufficient zinc levels are also important to minimize the effects of cadmium and copper toxicity.
- Zinc has also been reported to serve a vital role in the proper maintenance of the skeletal system, skin, hair, and nails, along with wound healing, appetite regulation and to stabilize mood.
- A zinc deficiency commonly causes alcoholic liver, fatigue, hypoglycemia and hypothyroidism. Other symptoms might include impotence, lack of taste and smell, birth defects, diabetes, failure to thrive, poor wound healing and prostate problems.
- Excessive zinc intakes may result in anemia, iron deficiency, nausea, depression, vomiting and diarrhea.

# Chapter 15 References

Metametrix Clinical Laboratory. 2015. Elements interpretive guide: blood, hair and urine.

# CHAPTER 16

# Boost Your Natural Detox Systems

## Detoxification Pathways

The human body has an amazingly elegant system for converting toxic compounds into a form that is harmless to the body and then eliminating it from the system altogether. While this natural detoxification process works well most of the time, in certain circumstances the body inadvertently makes relatively safe compounds toxic or it can increase the toxicity of already dangerous compounds. Therefore, understanding the process the body uses to eliminate the threat of environmental toxicants will be immensely helpful in your journey to improving your overall health.

As you probably already know, the liver is the chief agent in facilitation of all detoxification pathways in the body. Aided primarily by the kidneys, skin, and lungs—the liver is responsible for converting toxic compounds into a less toxic form so they can be eliminated.

The process of detoxifying toxic compounds is generally broken down into two phases, cleverly called Phase I and Phase II pathways. During Phase I, a series of enzymatic reactions are directed toward the toxicant in order to change its chemical nature to a form that is more easily removed from the system and that is less toxic at the same time. Phase II reactions, then, extend the work that has already been accomplished through the Phase I activity by adding additional chemical groups to the toxic compound. Generally, the purpose of Phase II reactions is to make the toxicants more water-soluble so they can more easily be eliminated in the urine or removed through the gastrointestinal tract.

When considering the detoxification pathways, there are ultimately two types of toxicants that you must think about: external toxicants that include toxic chemicals and heavy metals along with internal toxins that may be produced from bacteria, yeast or other microorganisms as well as the breakdown products that are normally produced through protein metabolism.

## External Toxicants

In addition to the heavy metals that have already been extensively discussed, there are other sources of external toxicants that you should consider for overall health. These include common chemicals such as volatile organic compounds (VOCs), solvents such as those used for cleaning, pesticides, herbicides, food additives, and even those compounds you are willingly exposed to such as medications and alcohol. Other insidious sources for external toxicants may include mold that causes "sick building syndrome" or even our modern "refined" diet which places an extreme burden on our liver due to the excessive consumption of sugar, high-fructose corn syrup, trans fatty acids, caffeine, alcohol, artificial sweeteners, genetically modified organisms, hidden antibiotics, environmental estrogens and other estrogenic compounds--along with the rampant use of plastics, which our systems can't break down or clear from the body.

## Internal Toxins

The gut is loaded with bacteria and yeast that produce waste products as a normal part of their daily metabolic functions. While some of these microorganisms are highly beneficial to our health, the pathological variety can produce cellular "debris" that wreaks havoc with our normal body functions by increasing inflammation and free radical production or oxidative stress. These "endotoxins" may even include carcinogenic compounds.

In addition to the toxins produced by pathogenic microorganisms, the normal metabolism of protein results in the production of byproducts that are potentially toxic if not properly detoxified, including urea and ammonia.

## Genetic and Hormonal Factors

There are individual differences between people that may affect their ability to properly deal with many of these toxic compounds.

These differences are often genetic polymorphisms in the detoxification enzymes that are critical for the Phase I and Phase II pathways. In a study looking at mice that were bred to be deficient in a protein important for transporting metals, known as metallothionein, an increase in the amount of weight gained over a lifetime was significantly higher than in mice with sufficient levels of metallothionein. In addition, the mice deficient in metallothionein were more sensitive to heavy metal exposure overall as well as to the effects of oxidative stress (Beattie et al. 1998).

Many heavy metals as well as environmental chemicals are known hormone disruptors—a common health consequence that cannot be adequately prevented through the normal detoxification pathways. What's more, it is thought that many of these toxicants cause problems with the regulation of hormones at extremely low levels—far below the EPA mandated "acceptable" level. These hormonal disturbances may interfere with the normal balance of sex hormones, thyroid hormones important for weight control, stress hormones and the hormones important for normal circadian rhythms (Hyman 2007).

*Assisting the Detoxification Pathways*

In order to be effective, the Phase I and Phase II detoxification pathways rely on a properly balanced diet that provides the appropriate ratio of fats, fiber, minerals, protein, phytochemicals and vitamins. For example, glutathione is a molecule that is critical for managing extreme oxidative insults and can easily become depleted when you are constantly being exposed to external and internal toxic compounds. The body requires an adequate supply of the essential amino acids in order to synthesize glutathione. Many phytochemicals in foods such as cruciferous vegetables, green tea, berries etc. can also increase the synthesis of enzymes required for the production of glutathione. The following table will get you started on ways to support your detoxification pathways.

Table 15. Tips for Supporting the Detoxification Pathways

| Minimize Exposure to Toxicants | Improve Elimination | Assist Gut Microflora | Supplement | Eat a Healthy Diet | Increase Fiber |
|---|---|---|---|---|---|
| Eat organic foods whenever possible | Aim for 1-2 healthy bowel movements daily | Consume freshly made fermented foods daily | Take a high potency multi-vitamin/mineral | Increase intake of cruciferous vegetables | Beans |
| Use a reverse osmosis or carbon filter for your drinking water | Drink at least 6-8 glasses of filtered water daily | Take a high quality probiotic supplement | Take 1000-4000 mg of Vitamin C daily | Eat raw garlic every day | Fruits |
| Use HEPA filters to purify air of daily living spaces | Exercise | Minimize the intake of sugar and gluten | Supplement with high quality omega-3 fatty acids | Increase bioflavonoid intake (berries, grapes, etc.) | Nuts |
| Regularly monitor for carbon monoxide and radon in your home | Utilize steam baths or saunas to increase sweating | | Consume natural chelators such as cilantro and chlorella | Try herbal detox teas such as dandelion, ginger, or burdock root | Vegetables |
| Remove allergens and dust from your home whenever possible | | | | Increase consumption of chlorophyll from green leafy vegetables | Seeds |

*The Importance of Glutathione*

The importance of glutathione in assisting with your natural detoxification process cannot be underestimated—particularly when you are talking about heavy metal toxicity. Whether or not you get sick (or even *how* sick you get) following an exposure to heavy metals or other environmental toxicants depends, in part, on how your body responds to the toxicant. Luckily, our bodies are equipped with the specialized innate detoxification system we've been describing, but it is not always functioning at optimal levels. Several factors can contribute to a sluggish detoxification system, including chronic inflammation and a genetic predisposition.

Glutathione plays a critical role in the Phase II reactions of the detoxification pathway and requires a number of "assistants" including many enzymes, other antioxidants and proteins that can transport molecules throughout the body. A genetic disposition for a sluggish detoxification system, along with constant exposure to toxicants, a poor diet and (unfortunately) old age can diminish the ability of glutathione and its helpers to properly do their jobs. Mercury, in particular, is known to deplete the body's supply of glutathione. Supplementation with glutathione and the molecules required by the body for its synthesis can help, but ultimately a better strategy is to improve your body's ability to fine-tune the glutathione system on its own. In order for your glutathione system to work efficiently, your body requires three key elements (Mercola 2013):

- *A supply of glutathione to the cells*
- *An enzyme known as glutathione s-transferase, which is important for glutathione to convert toxicants into less dangerous forms*
- *Transport proteins that can move the glutathione-transformed toxicants out of your body*

Strategies for increasing the glutathione available for use in your body as well as the supporting enzymes and transport proteins can include dietary changes as well as specialized supplementation. Consuming foods that are high in the amino acid cysteine, which is a primary component of glutathione, can naturally increase glutathione levels. Excellent sources of cysteine include high quality whey, poultry, eggs and non-GMO soy.

Once your glutathione levels have been boosted, the enzymes and transport proteins that are critical for glutathione to do its job can be supported through the consumption of "superfoods." Glutathione is a sulfur-containing molecule, therefore foods that are high in sulfur such as cruciferous vegetables. In addition, other supplements that are known to activate the detoxification system can be taken, including (Mercola 2013):

- *Fruit extracts from Terminalia chebula—known to have anti-inflammatory properties and upregulation of natural antioxidants within the body*
- *R-Lipoic Acid—A potent chelator of copper and natural antioxidant*
- *Lumbrokinase—an agent that is extracted from earth worms that dissolves fibrin and assists with healthy blood flow*
- *Pine Bark Extract—Supports the activity of Vitamin C*

## Detoxification Support

Committing to a program for detoxing your body of heavy metals is a great start toward regaining your health. In addition to the program that you and your doctor design to best assist your recovery, there are certain things you can do on a day-to-day basis that will also help in the removal of heavy metals. Following are some simple suggestions for everyday items that you can use right now!

- **Cilantro:** Also known as coriander, cilantro is a popular herb in many ethnic dishes and it is also a natural chelating agent for heavy metals (Omura and Beckman 1995)!
- **Chlorella:** Also known as blue green algae, chlorella is a supplement that has been shown to be effective in assisting the detoxification and removal of heavy metals from the body.
- **Bentonite Clay:** Toxic compounds will commonly adhere to bentonite clay, which is a form of volcanic ash, through a process called adsorption. High-grade forms of bentonite can

be consumed orally and have been particularly useful in the removal of lead and cadmium (Meneguin et al.).

- **Selenium:** An essential mineral in small concentrations, selenium must be taken with caution (preferable on the advice of a health care practitioner). Maintaining adequate selenium levels in the body is especially useful for aiding your body in the elimination of mercury (Patrick 2009).

- **Garlic:** A well-known antioxidant, garlic is also helpful in aiding the elimination of heavy metals from the body. Garlic is particularly useful to assist in the removal of cadmium from the body (Cha 1987).

- **Milk Thistle:** Milk thistle may be used as a supportive agent during the process of removing heavy metals from the body. Known to be a significant supportive agent for the liver, flavonoids in milk thistle have also been shown to have potent antioxidant properties (Abenavoli et al. 2010).

- **Turmeric:** Turmeric may be a useful supplement for reducing the effects of heavy metal exposure. Studies have shown a reduction in the toxic effects from arsenic exposure (Pantazis et al. 2010). Turmeric is also known to have potent antioxidant properties, which may be the primary reason it has so many beneficial uses in the detoxification process (Bengmark, Mesa, and Gil 2009).

- **Zeolite:** Zeolite is basically volcanic ash that is primarily a "potassium-calcium-sodium-aluminosilicate." It has been described as having tiny "cage-like" structures that are ideal for trapping heavy metals. Once the heavy metals have been contained within the zeolite cage, they can safely be excreted from the body.

- **Himalayan Shilajit Extract (Asphaltum punjabinum):** Is a purified form of shilajit. This is a naturally occurring phytocomplex found in high mountain rocks, especially those in the Himalayas and Hindu Kush ranges of the Indian subcontinent. It is formed from decomposed plant material that has been preserved in the dark pressure of rocky crevasses. As the sun warms the rocks and the snow melts, the shilajit seeps out and is scraped from the stone by hand. It is composed mainly of humic substances including fulvic acid and trace elements.

- **N–Acetyl–L–Cysteine (NAC):** Exposure to heavy metals increases free radical production and oxidative stress. NAC reacts with reactive oxygen species (ROS) and stimulates the body to produce glutathione. This enhances cell survival after toxin exposure.
- **Vitamin C:** Vitamin C is an ideal detoxer, antioxidant and an all–purpose nutrient. It supports collagen synthesis and the stabilized (excellent) forms offer significant reactive oxygen species (ROS) inhibition without irritating the gastrointestinal tract.
- **R–Lipoic Acid (RLA):** RLA is an excellent antioxidant and most important for the mitochondrial function. It improves energy production, and protects the mitochondria from damage. It is very important in recycling Vitamin C, Glutathione, Coenzyme Q10, Tocopherols (part of Vitamin E), reduces DNA damage and helps the brain work better. It also aids in weight loss and blood sugar control.

Use of these agents can help support your body during the detoxification process. An important thing to consider while detoxing (under any protocol) is an adverse reaction to toxins that are released into the body during the detox process that is commonly referred to as the Jarisch–Herxheimer reaction. Originally described in syphilis patients undergoing treatment with penicillin, it is widely recognized to occur any time the body is quickly eliminated hazardous elements from the system. If this happens to you, be patient—the initial feeling will eventually pass and your symptoms will then improve rapidly.

If you are still unsure if your symptoms could be due to heavy metal toxicity, the following table is an easy guide to symptoms of some of the most toxic of all the heavy metals.

Table 16. Symptoms and sources of the most common toxic heavy metals (adapted in part with permission from Genova/Metametrix Clinical Laboratory (2015))

|  | Common Symptoms | Common Sources |
|---|---|---|
| **Mercury** | • Mental difficulties<br>• Tremor<br>• Gastrointestinal disturbances<br>• Kidney disturbances<br>• Gingivitis<br>• Poor immunity | • Dental amalgams<br>• Fish consumption<br>• Preservatives<br>• Vaccines<br>• Industrial practices |
| **Lead** | • Anemia<br>• Kidney disturbances<br>• High blood pressure<br>• Loss of appetite<br>• Muscle pain<br>• Constipation<br>• Metallic taste<br>• Lowered IQ in children | • Home remedies<br>• Lead-based paint<br>• Contaminated soil<br>• Lead plumbing |
| **Arsenic** | • Blackfoot disease<br>• Diarrhea<br>• Protein in the urine<br>• Dark pigments on the skin<br>• Garlic breath | • Drinking water<br>• Seafood<br>• Glues<br>• Industrial exposure<br>• Contaminated supplements<br>• Cigarette smoke<br>• Arsenic-treated wood<br>• Processed chicken |
| **Aluminum** | • Abnormal speech<br>• Alzheimer's disease<br>• Parkinson's disease<br>• Abnormal bone formation<br>• Jerky movement | • Aluminum cookware<br>• Antacids<br>• Drinking water<br>• Tobacco<br>• Marijuana smoke |
| **Cadmium** | • Bone pain<br>• Low back pain<br>• Low bone density<br>• Kidney disturbances<br>• High blood pressure<br>• Vascular disease | • Industrial practices<br>• Spray paint<br>• Tobacco smoke<br>• Car emissions<br>• Plants grown in cadmium-rich soil |

Table 17. Comprehensive list of sources for the most common toxic heavy metals (adapted in part with permission from Genova/Metametrix Clinical Laboratory (2015))

| Source Type | Mercury | Lead | Arsenic | Cadmium | Aluminum |
|---|---|---|---|---|---|
| **Cosmetics** | • Calomel (body powder, talc)<br>• Skin lightening creams<br>• Tattooing | • Some red lipsticks<br>• Toothpaste | | | • Antiperspirants<br>• Toothpaste |
| **Food** | • Predator fish | • Canned fruit and juices<br>• Box wine<br>• Bone meal<br>• Organ meats<br>• Lead-capped wine bottles | • Drinking water<br>• Seawater<br>• Well water<br>• Seafood<br>• Chicken | • Drinking water<br>• Soft water<br>• Water from galvanized plumbing<br>• Refined wheat flour<br>• Canned evaporated milk<br>• Processed foods<br>• Oysters, kidney, liver | • Baking powder<br>• Soda cans<br>• Drinking water<br>• Milk processed with aluminum equipment<br>• Pickled foods<br>• FD&C color additives<br>• Vanilla powder<br>• Table salt, seasonings<br>• Bleached flour<br>• American cheese |
| **Industrial related** | • Adhesives<br>• Photo-engraving<br>• Sewage sludge | | • Automobile exhaust<br>• Wood preserves<br>• Sewage disposal | • Electroplates<br>• Polyvinyl plastics<br>• Nickel-cadmium batteries<br>• Rust-proofing materials | • Automobile exhaust |

| | Column 1 | Column 2 | Column 3 | Column 4 | Column 5 |
|---|---|---|---|---|---|
| **Medical related** | • Dental Amalgams<br>• Thimerosal<br>• Laxatives<br>• Hemorrhoid suppositories<br>• Merthiolate<br>• Psoriasis ointments | • Certain herbal preps | | • Dental appliances | • Antacids<br>• Nasal spray<br>• Dental Amalgams<br>• Aluminum silicate<br>• Sutures |
| **Household** | • Broken thermometers<br>• Solvent-thinned paints<br>• Fabric Softeners<br>• Floor waxes and polishes<br>• Air conditioner filters<br>• Some batteries<br>• Fluorescent (energy-efficient) light bulbs | • Some toys<br>• Lead house paint<br>• Drinking water from lead plumbing<br>• Improperly glazed pottery<br>• Painted glassware<br>• Pencils<br>• Utensils<br>• Curtain weights<br>• Putty<br>• Car batteries | • Rat poison<br>• Detergents<br>• Colored chalk<br>• Wallpaper dye and plaster | • Ceramic glazes<br>• Paint pigments<br>• Silver polish<br>• Rubber carpet backing | • Cooling utensils<br>• Ceramics<br>• Rat poison |
| **Ag- related** | • Methylmercury fungicide-treated grains<br>• Wood preservatives<br>• Fungicides | • Some Vegetables<br>• Lead-arsenate pesticides<br>• Tobacco | • Insecticide residues<br>• Wine | • Tobacco<br>• Phosphate fertilizers | |
| **Other** | • Leather tanning products | • Rain water and snow<br>• Newsprint<br>• Color prints<br>• Lead shot | | | |

# Chapter 16 References

Abenavoli, L., R. Capasso, N. Milic, and F. Capasso. 2010. "Milk thistle in liver diseases: past, present, future." *Phytotherapy research: PTR* 24 (10):1423-32. doi: 10.1002/ptr.3207.

Beattie, J. H., A. M. Wood, A. M. Newman, I. Bremner, K. H. Choo, A. E. Michalska, J. S. Duncan, and P. Trayhurn. 1998. "Obesity and hyperleptinemia in metallothionein (-I and -II) null mice." *Proceedings of the National Academy of Sciences of the United States of America* 95 (1):358-63.

Bengmark, S., M. D. Mesa, and A. Gil. 2009. "Plant-derived health: the effects of turmeric and curcuminoids." *Nutricion hospitalaria* 24 (3):273-81.

Metametrix Clinical Laboratory. 2015. Elements interpretive guide: blood, hair and urine.

Cha, C. W. 1987. "A study on the effect of garlic to the heavy metal poisoning of rat." *Journal of Korean medical science* 2 (4):213-24.

Hyman, M. 2007. "Systems biology, toxins, obesity, and functional medicine." 13th International symposium of The Institute for Functional Medicine.

Meneguin, J.G., G.R. Luz, I.C. Ostroski, A.S. Dornellas de Barros, and M.L. Gimenes. Maringa.

Mercola, J. 2013. "Revised protocol for detoxifying your body from mercury exposure." Accessed December 1, 2014. articles.mercola. com/sites/articles/archive/2013/01/13/mercury-detoxification-protocol.aspx.

Omura, Y., and S. L. Beckman. 1995. "Role of mercury (Hg) in resistant infections & effective treatment of Chlamydia trachomatis and Herpes family viral infections (and potential treatment for cancer) by removing localized Hg deposits with Chinese parsley and delivering effective antibiotics using various drug uptake enhancement methods." *Acupuncture & electro-therapeutics research* 20 (3-4):195-229.

Pantazis, P., A. Varman, C. Simpson-Durand, J. Thorpe, S. Ramalingam, D. Subramaniam, C. Houchen, M. Ihnat, S. Anant, and R. P. Ramanujam. 2010. "Curcumin and turmeric attenuate arsenic-induced angiogenesis in ovo." *Alternative therapies in health and medicine* 16 (2):12-4.

Patrick, K. 2009. "Selenium helps remove mercury from the body." Natural News Accessed October 28, 2014. http://www. naturalnews.com/026729_selenium_mercury_fish.html.

# CHAPTER 17

# Boost Your Overall Health

## What You Should Know About Going "Organic"

You may have heard about a recent study published by Stanford University comparing organic versus conventional foods that came up with the following conclusions:·

The published literature lacks strong evidence that organic foods are significantly more nutritious than conventional foods. Consumption of organic foods may reduce exposure to pesticide residues and antibiotic-resistant bacteria (Smith-Spangler et al. 2012).

There are several problems with this study, including the fact that it does not mention differences in key vitamins and minerals that have already been shown to be present in higher levels in organic versus conventional foods. However, the bigger problem is the implication that there is no nutritional difference between foods containing pesticide residues and antibiotic-resistant bacteria and foods without! If we examine those two issues alone, it becomes quickly evident that both consumption of pesticides and exposure to antibiotic resistant bacteria can pose significant health hazards.

*Health Effects from Pesticide Exposure*

The Environmental Protection Agency has an ongoing evaluation program that estimates the carcinogenic potential for the various pesticides that present an exposure risk in the environment. In order to make these risk assessments, EPA officials evaluate all of the most current "peer-reviewed" literature available, including laboratory animal findings, studies on the effects of pesticides on metabolism, structural relationships with other known carcinogens, and, when available human epidemiology studies (Environmental Protection Agency 2014). Evaluation of the EPA results demonstrates that 30 percent of all insecticides, 60 percent of all herbicides, and 90 percent of all fungicides may be carcinogenic (Mercola 2013a). Even worse, all of these chemicals are used on conventional farms, where they may easily contaminate the fruits and vegetables that will ultimately end up on your plate.

Cancer concerns may be the most frightening risk for exposure to pesticides, but there are other adverse health effects that can be equally devastating. Environmental chemicals can often wreak havoc with steroid hormones—including those that affect development of the reproductive system. One study that examined three common antifungal agents used in agriculture found that two of the three agents reduced testosterone levels in both adult and newborn rats by 40-68 percent! When the researchers conducted further studies to see how these results might translate to human health, they discovered that all THREE of the antifungal agents decreased the steroid hormones, including estradiol, progesterone and testosterone (Goetz et al. 2009).

While it is impossible to completely avoid exposure to pesticides that are used so frequently in the environment where we live, we can minimize exposure through the consumption of "organically-labeled" foods whenever possible. In addition, you can effectively clean your fruits and vegetables by washing them in a mixture of white vinegar and water or a similar commercial "veggie wash" product before eating them.

The Environmental Working Group (EWG) is an organization that monitors many environmental health issues, including the presence of pesticide residues on conventionally grown foods. They frequently publish lists of foods that tend to be extremely contaminated with pesticides, and alternatively, foods that are generally low in pesticide residues. This is very useful information because it allows you to maximize the safety of your food supply within a modest budget by being selective in the foods that you buy "organic"—which tend to be more expensive. The following table lists the most recent results from the Environmental Working Group's results (Environmental Working Group 2014):

Table 18. Results from the Environmental Working Group's examination of pesticide residues on the most commonly purchased fruits and vegetables (EWG 2014)

| "Dirty Dozen" Fruits and Vegetables | "Clean 15" Fruits and Vegetables |
|:---:|:---:|
| Apples | Avocadoes |
| Strawberries | Sweet corn |
| Grapes | Pineapple |
| Celery | Cabbage |
| Peaches | Frozen sweet peas |
| Spinach | Onions |
| Sweet bell peppers | Asparagus |
| Imported nectarines | Mangoes |
| Cucumbers | Papayas |
| Cherry tomatoes | Kiwi |
| Imported snap peas | Eggplant |
| Potatoes | Grapefruit |
| | Cantaloupe |
| | Cauliflower |
| | Sweet potatoes |

*Exposure to Antibiotic Resistant Bacteria*

Antimicrobial resistance is currently one of the most urgent problems within the realm of conventional medicine. The microbial pathogens that are the target for antimicrobial agents, most notably antibiotics, tend to be extremely adaptive. They reproduce rapidly and therefore can change and adapt in response to environmental conditions at a rapid rate. As a consequence, when these pathogens are exposed to reagents such as commonly used antibiotics, a percentage of them are not killed and over time, these "resistant" few become the dominant form. Fairly rapidly, antimicrobial agents that were once very effective become relatively useless. The spread of these resistant forms then perpetuates the problem.

If you contract an infection with a microbial resistant pathogen, it may prolong the time you spend being sick, increase the associated costs and increase your risk of death. In fact, the death rate for individuals who contract serious infections, usually within a hospital setting, are twice as likely to die than someone who has an infection with a non-resistant form of the same bacteria (World Health Organization 2014). For example, you are 64 percent more likely to die if you contract a resistant form of the *Staphylococcus* bacteria known as MRSA (**m**ethicillin-**r**esistant *Staphylococcus aureus*) than if you are infected with a non-resistant form of Staph.

A few of the most publicized diseases that are at the highest risk due to the emergence of microbial resistant pathogens include: Gonorrhea (if untreated, may cause infertility, failed pregnancies and neonatal blindness), *Staphylococcus aureus,* intestinal pathogens, tuberculosis, HIV and malaria.

According to the World Health Organization, antibiotic resistance poses a risk to our health in many ways, including the prevention of effective treatment for infections caused by many bacteria, viruses and fungi (Mercola 2014). Antibiotic resistance is also present globally, with approximately 450,000 new cases of the resistant tuberculosis strain alone (Mercola 2014). Antibiotic resistance is jeopardizing our ability to treat tropical diseases such as malaria to more ordinary urinary tract infections. In some cases, previously treated diseases such as Gonorrhea may soon fall in the category of 'untreatable'. Antibiotic resistance also presents a significant strain on resources, as health care costs soar.

## Increasing Incidence of Colon Cancer in People Under 50

There is a disturbing trend in the incidence of colon cancer in this country that may be predictive of other types of cancers and possible other diseases that have been traditionally considered to be associated with "old age." Increased screening in people over the age of 50 has resulted in the slow decline in the incidence of colon cancer since the 1980's. However, a recent study on people under the age of 50 showed a disturbing increase in the rate of colon cancer among this population (Bailey et al. 2014). What's more, the colon cancer detected in this younger population tends to be more advanced and aggressive than that seen in older people. At this point, the reasons for this trend are purely speculative, but it isn't hard to imagine given the diet and vast array of environmental exposures that young people are submitted to from birth—or even before birth. If this trend continues into other areas of medicine, the ravages of old age may start for many of us well before our time.

## Maintaining Good Gastrointestinal Health

The new buzz in research circles describes the gastrointestinal tract as the "new, last frontier," "the second brain," "the gateway to health" and other equally descriptive terms. Considering that the vast majority of genetic material (90 percent) found in our bodies is not human, but microbial DNA—it is no wonder. While a healthy gut is vital for the proper synthesis and absorption of many vitamins and minerals and plays a key role in modulating our immune system, an imbalance can cause equally devastating conditions that range from severe gastrointestinal disorders such as Crohns and IBS to neurological conditions like depression. A short-list of the more severe diseases linked to an unhealthy gut includes autism spectrum disorder, chronic fatigue syndrome, diabetes, obesity and rheumatoid arthritis. Heavy metal toxicity is a "key player" for damaging the GI system, which leads to "leaky gut" and malabsorption issues. Unfortunately, modern society subscribes to a number of common practices that do not lend themselves to maintaining a healthy gut, including (Kresser 2014):

- Use of common medications (antibiotics, birth control, NSAIDs, etc.)
- Typical standard American diet (lots of refined carbohydrates, sugar and processed foods)
- Low consumption of fermentable fibers
- Unhealthy dietary components such as wheat and industrial seed oils
- Chronic stress
- Chronic infections

One of the primary consequences of a living an unhealthy lifestyle is the development of what is commonly termed "leaky gut syndrome." This is a condition where the lining of the gastrointestinal tract becomes damaged in such a way that it can no longer provide an adequate barrier between the "unwanted" components within the gut and the delicate systems within your body. In some cases, proteins that are much larger than normal are absorbed into the blood stream causing the body to launch an immune reaction in response because it fails to recognize the proteins as "normal." Data is accumulating to suggest that this sequence of events may play a fundamental role in the development of autoimmune diseases.

One of the most effective ways to improve your overall gut health is to first, get tested for heavy metal toxicity; then detoxify and get back to the basics, by consuming more traditionally fermented foods and taking excellent probiotics. Many fermented foods are excellent sources of vital nutrients such as vitamin K2, many B vitamins and of course as natural sources of probiotics. A few of the healthiest fermented foods include kefir and yogurt made from unpasteurized milk (which changes the structure of the milk proteins), cheese curd, Japanese natto, and fermented vegetables such as homemade sauerkraut and kimchi. In addition, heavy metal exposure can wreak havoc on the ecosystem of the gastrointestinal tract; yet fermented foods contain a wide variety of natural chelating agents, making them a good source for detoxing as well as improving gut health.

Once you have incorporated fermented foods into your diet, you can continue on the path to a healthy digestive system by avoiding sugar sources as much as possible. The pathogenic bacteria, yeast and fungi that can quickly overtake the beneficial bugs in your gut LOVE sugar. This, along with the spikes in blood sugar levels due to sugar's impact on insulin can cause serious health effects.

Improving your gut health will go a long way toward acquiring a healthy immune and nervous system as well. Very few people realize that 80 percent of our immune system is actually located in the gut. When you look at it from that perspective it is easy to understand why so many people with autoimmune and other inflammatory conditions also have digestive problems. In fact, it is becoming more and more understood that a healthy gut is your number ONE defense against all diseases (once you have removed other toxicants such as heavy metals!).

Needless to say, one of the most direct paths toward a healthy immune system is through the adequate care of your digestive tract. A flourishing inner ecosystem will provide a strong defense against many types of environmental insults and help you find your way toward drastic improvements in your overall health.

## The Perils of Processed Foods

Processed foods tend to have high levels of food additives such as nitrites/nitrates, potassium bromate, propyl paraben, butylated hydroxyanisole, butylated hydroxytoluene, propyl gallate, theobromine, artificial flavors, artificial colors, diacetyl, phosphate additives, aluminum additives and the list goes on. However, the environmental working group recognizes these 12 additives as the "dirty dozen" of food additives that should be actively avoided.

*Nitrates and Nitrites*

You will find nitrites and nitrates in many types of cured meats, including bacon, hot dogs and salami. They serve as preservatives; however, they react with a component of your proteins known as amines—forming nitrosamines. Unfortunately, nitrosamines are known cancer-causing agents. Links have been discovered between nitrosamines and stomach cancer, esophageal cancer and possibly brain and thyroid cancers. It is interesting to note, however, that although some green leafy vegetables such as spinach are naturally high in nitrates, no association with cancer from ingesting these foods has been found (IARC 2010).

*Potassium Bromate*

Potassium bromate is a food additive used in the baking process of bread and other flour-based products such as crackers—even though it is recognized as a carcinogen by the state of California. Even though baking is thought to convert the majority of potassium bromate to a non-carcinogenic form, some toxic residue may still remain. Interestingly, the United States still allows the addition of potassium bromate to flour, even though it is prohibited in the United Kingdom, Canada and the European Union.

*Propyl Paraben*

The FDA uses an interesting method of classifying potentially toxic food additives as "generally recognized as safe" or GRAS, even though many of them are far from it. Propyl paraben is a perfect example of a GRAS food additive that has been shown to cause disturbing health effects in animal studies. A confirmed endocrine-disrupting compound, propyl paraben decreases sperm count and testosterone levels in rats (Oishi 2002). In addition to affecting male fertility, propyl paraben shows weak estrogenic activity and may worsen breast cancer (Okubo et al. 2001) and infertility in women (Smith et al. 2013). In 2010, a study conducted by the U.S. federal government detected propyl paraben in the urine of 91 percent of Americans tested (Calafat et al. 2010).

*Butylated Hydroxyanisole*

Butylated hydroxyanisole (BHA) is another GRAS food additive even though it is "reasonably anticipated to be a human carcinogen" by the National Toxicology Program and "possible human carcinogen" by the International Cancer Agency.

In addition to its probable cancer-causing effects, BHA is also an endocrine disruptor known to decrease fertility and thyroid hormones in rats (Jeong et al. 2005). Studies done in rats also suggest that BHA may also cause developmental disorders, increased infant mortality and behavioral disorders in adolescents.

*Butylated Hydroxytoluene*

Butylated hydroxytoluene (BHT) is chemically similar to BHA, and like BHA is an FDA-designated GRAS compound that is allowed to be added as a preservative to our food. In fact, BHT and BHA are often used together due to their "complementary" activities.

While BHT is not a classified carcinogen like BHA, some animal studies have developed tumors following exposure to BHT. There is also evidence to suggest that BHT may act as an endocrine disruptor as well.

*Propyl Gallate*

Propyl gallate is typically used as a food preservative in products that contain edible fats. Propyl gallate is an FDA-designated GRAS even though there are health concerns associated with its safety. While the research is inconclusive at this point, some studies have suggested that propyl gallate may contribute to brain cancers and infertility.

*Theobromine*

Theobromine is an alkaloid with effects similar to caffeine that was independently labeled as GRAS outside of the FDA's approval! Animal studies have raised concern regarding reproductive and development issues caused by theobromine, which is found in chocolate and added to a variety of foods such as bread, cereal and many sport drinks.

*Artificial Flavors*

Artificial flavoring is an extremely common item listed in the ingredients of processed foods. According to the Environmental Working group it is the fourth more frequently food ingredient following salt, sugar and water. What's more, the term "natural flavor" appears on one out of every seven labels as a food additive! This terminology is intentionally ambiguous and can be used to describe many questionable chemicals that may be added to your food! Many of these "natural flavor" ingredients can contain very unnatural ingredients such as propylene glycol and BHA that are categorized as incidental additives and therefore do not require disclosure by the FDA. The most disturbing aspect of this use of food additives is the "secrecy" involved—which prevents concerned consumers from the right to choose whether or not they want to consume them.

*Artificial Colors*

Aside from the arguably unethical use of artificial colors to increase the appeal of foods that otherwise lack any nutritional value, safety concerns have been raised about their safety. The tumor-causing compounds known as 4-methylimidazole and furan have been found as contaminants of several artificial coloring agents. Furthermore, ongoing debates on the effects of artificial colors on children's behavior have raised concern about their frequent use in foods that are marketed toward kids.

*Phosphate Additives*

Despite being associated with heart disease and death, phosphates are commonly used as food additives. They are found in a range of products from baked goods to meat products and are particularly common in highly processed foods and fast food.

*Aluminum Additives*

Despite the alarming accumulation of data implicating aluminum in a range of diseases from Alzheimer's to heart disease, sodium aluminum phosphate and sodium aluminum sulfate, are commonly used as stabilizers in a variety of processed foods! Please see table 19 for classification of the most common food additives.

Table 19. Common FDA-approved food additives (adapted from FDA. gov 2013)

| Food Additive | Purpose | Typical Product Labels |
| --- | --- | --- |
| **Preservatives** | Antimicrobial; Antioxidant (preserves "freshness") | Ascorbic acid, citric acid, sodium benzoate, calcium propionate, sodium erythorbate, sodium nitrite, calcium sorbate, potassium sorbate, BHA, BHT, EDTA, tocopherols (Vitamin E) |
| **Sweeteners** | Adds sweetness (may be with or without extra calories) | Sucrose (sugar), glucose, fructose, sorbitol, mannitol, corn syrup, high fructose corn syrup, saccharin, aspartame, sucralose, acesulfame potassium (acesulfame-K), neotame |

| | | |
|---|---|---|
| **Color Additives** | Offset effects of photobleaching; correct variations in color that naturally occur; enhance natural coloring of food; provide color to colorless and "fun" foods | FD&C Blue Nos. 1 and 2, FD&C Green No. 3, FD&C Red Nos. 3 and 40, FD&C Yellow Nos. 5 and 6, Orange B, Citrus Red No. 2, annatto extract, beta-carotene, grape skin extract, cochineal extract or carmine, paprika oleoresin, caramel color, fruit and vegetable juices, saffron (Note: Exempt color additives are not required to be declared by name on labels but may be declared simply as colorings or color added) |
| **Flavors and Spices** | Add specific flavors (may be natural or synthetic) | Natural flavoring, artificial flavor, and spices |
| **Flavor Enhancers** | Enhance natural flavors | Monosodium glutamate (MSG), hydrolyzed soy protein, autolyzed yeast extract, disodium guanylate or inosinate |
| **Fat Replacers** | Provide expected texture and a creamy "mouth-feel" in reduced-fat foods | Olestra, cellulose gel, carrageenan, polydextrose, modified food starch, microparticulated egg white protein, guar gum, xanthan gum, whey protein concentrate |
| **Nutrients** | Replace nutrients lost during "processing" and add nutrients that may be lacking in the diet | Thiamine hydrochloride, riboflavin (Vitamin B₂), niacin, niacinamide, folate or folic acid, beta carotene, potassium iodide, iron or ferrous sulfate, alpha tocopherols, ascorbic acid, Vitamin D, amino acids (L-tryptophan, L-lysine, L-leucine, L-methionine) |

| | | |
|---|---|---|
| **Emulsifiers** | Allow smooth mixing of ingredients, prevent separation | Soy lecithin, mono- and diglycerides, egg yolks, polysorbates, sorbitan monostearate |
| | Keep emulsified products stable, reduce stickiness, control crystallization, keep ingredients dispersed, and to help products dissolve more easily | |
| **Stabilizers and Thickeners, Binders, Texturizers** | Produce uniform texture, improve "mouth-feel" | Gelatin, pectin, guar gum, carrageenan, xanthan gum, whey |
| **pH Control Agents and acidulants** | Control acidity and alkalinity, prevent spoilage | Lactic acid, citric acid, ammonium hydroxide, sodium carbonate |
| **Leavening Agents** | Promote rising of baked goods | Baking soda, monocalcium phosphate, calcium carbonate |
| **Anti-caking agents** | Keep powdered foods free-flowing, prevent moisture absorption | Calcium silicate, iron ammonium citrate, silicon dioxide |
| **Humectants** | Retain moisture | Glycerin, sorbitol |
| **Yeast Nutrients** | Promote growth of yeast | Calcium sulfate, ammonium phosphate |
| **Dough Strengtheners and Conditioners** | Produce more stable dough | Ammonium sulfate, azodicarbonamide, L-cysteine |
| **Firming Agents** | Maintain crispness and firmness | Calcium chloride, calcium lactate |
| **Enzyme Preparations** | Modify proteins, polysaccharides and fats | Enzymes, lactase, papain, rennet, chymosin |
| **Gases** | Serve as propellant, aerate, or create carbonation | Carbon dioxide, nitrous oxide |

# Vitamins, Minerals and "Other" Supplementation

In addition to supplementing the essential minerals discussed in Chapter 16, there are other important nutrients that can make a significant contribution to your overall health. Here will discuss some of the most highly recommended supplements as well as the importance of acquiring all the essential vitamins.

*Probiotics*

Before the days of refrigeration and processed food with long shelf lives, people had to find natural ways of preserving their food from day to day. One common practice included the art of food fermentation. Fermented foods were not only safe to eat for longer periods of time--they contained a wealth of beneficial microbes that helped repopulate the good bacteria in the gut on a continual basis. Today, we know that these beneficial microbes are part of the foundation for good health. Unfortunately, we no longer consume fermented foods on a regular (or even semi-regular) basis. In addition, overuse of antibiotics, environmental pollutants, stress and poor nutrition contribute to the decline in microbial populations of the gut. One way to counteract this unfortunate situation is by supplementing with a high quality source of probiotics.

A condition that is increasingly recognized as causing significant gastrointestinal problems is overgrowth of bacteria in the small intestine, known as small intestine bacteria overgrowth (SIBO). While it is extremely important to maintain the proper balance of good bacteria in the large intestine, the bacterial populations of the small intestine are generally kept very low. The presence of these bacteria in the small intestine can interfere with the proper absorption of nutrients and can damage the gut lining. Treatment generally involves the use of antibiotics followed by a very strict diet, including the Specific Carbohydrate Diet, Gut and Psychology Syndrome Diet, Low Fodmap Diet, Cedars-Sinai Diet, or a combination of the above (refer to the resources section at the end of the book for more information).

*Resveratrol*

Resveratrol is a potent antioxidant that has been referred to as the "fountain of youth" because of its extensive list of beneficial properties. The long list of resveratrol benefits includes anti-cancer properties, reversal of oxidative stress, anti-inflammatory properties, improvement of lipid profiles, cardio- and neuro-protective properties, and anti-diabetic activities (Mercola 2013b). However, the benefits don't just stop there, resveratrol also has broad-spectrum antimicrobial activity!

Resveratrol can be found in a number of natural food sources such as berries, cacao, the skin of red grapes, peanuts, pomegranates and red wine.

*Ubiquinol*

Ubiquinol is the reduced form of coenzyme Q10, which is the form that your body uses in every oxygen-requiring system of the body! Cellular organelles called mitochondria are the body's tiny "power houses"—converting energy from food into ATP, which is the form used by cells in the body. A deficiency in ubiquinol impairs the mitochondria's ability to function properly and prevents proper synthesis and distribution of ATP to the rest of the body, including the all-important heart muscles, brain and liver. If that is not enough to convince you of the importance of ubiquinol for optimal health, then consider that impairment of the mitochondria is associated with accelerated aging and many age-related diseases.

*Vitamin A*

Vitamin A is a term given to a group of fat-soluble retinoid compounds that are important for cellular communication, proper immune function, reproduction and vision (Health). Vitamin A that comes from the diet occurs either in a preformed version (i.e. retinol and retinyl ester) or as the "provitamin" A carotenoid (such as beta-carotene). A provitamin is an inactive form that is converted by the body into the active form. Preformed vitamin A is primarily found in foods from animal sources, such as dairy, fish and meat. Provitamin A, such as beta-carotene, is primarily found in plant pigments.

*Vitamin B*

There are a number of essential forms of "vitamin B" that includes vitamin B12 and the various vitamins B6.

Vitamin B12 is critical for a number of important pathways within the body such as the proper formation of red blood cells, neurological function and the synthesis of DNA. Vitamin B12 is also critical in the synthesis of the essential amino acid methionine, which is important for the proper function of DNA, RNA, lipids, hormones and many proteins. Vitamin B12 also plays a vital role in the metabolism of fat and protein metabolism as well as hemoglobin synthesis (World Health Organization 2014). Natural sources of vitamin B12 include animal and dairy products, but are generally not found in plant foods.

When you see "vitamin B6," it generally refers to a group of six different compounds, including: pyridoxine, pyridoxal, pyridoxamine and the ester version of those three parent compounds. Vitamin B6 functions as a "coenzyme" in the body that is primarily involved in protein metabolism, neurotransmitter biosynthesis and homocysteine regulation (National Institutes of Health 2014). Vitamin B6 is most abundantly found in animal products, starchy vegetables and non-citrus fruits.

It is important to remember that two very common polymorphisms in the MTHFR gene are found among Americans. These gene variants prevent you from utilizing the active form of folate and can result in a bad reaction to folic acid supplements. If you have been diagnosed as having one of the common mutations, you may consider eating more green leafy vegetables or other food sources or supplementing with a methylated form, such as l-methylfolate.

*Vitamin C*

Linus Pauling, the only American scientist to receive two unshared Nobel prizes (one in 1954 for chemistry and the Nobel peace prize in 1962), argued that Vitamin C is one of the most important essential substances known. Unfortunately, before his death in 1994 he became a source of ridicule by the medical establishment for what was considered to be "wild" claims about the importance of this essential nutrient. Today, Linus Pauling would be smiling because increasingly the evidence is supporting his views on the critical nature of Vitamin

C to our health and disease status. Needless to say, vitamin C is an incredibly important essential nutrient for human health. Whereas most animals can synthesize vitamin C, humans are alone in their need to consume 100 percent of their requirements through the diet. Vitamin C is known to be an important ingredient for the biosynthesis of collagen, which is a necessary component of connective tissue. In addition, vitamin C is involved in the biosynthesis of L-carnitine, some neurotransmitters and protein metabolism. One of the best-known roles for vitamin C in the body is that of an antioxidant. A lack of vitamin C causes a disease known as scurvy, which results in symptoms of gum disease, generalized weakness and anemia.

Ongoing research into the use of vitamin C as an adjunct therapy for cancer patients to lower the side effects associated with treatment and to improve overall quality of life has shown significant promise. Additionally, high dose vitamin C is thought to be an effective agent against many infectious diseases.

*Vitamin D*

Increasingly, experts believe that deficiencies in vitamin D are linked to the severe decline observed in overall health around the world. Some estimates suggest that as many as 85 percent of all people have a vitamin D deficiency (Mercola 2014).

The importance of serum vitamin D levels in cancer has been shown in multiple studies and appears to affect the development of as many as 16 different types of cancer (Mercola 2014)! What's more, a recent meta-analysis looking at 56 different randomized trials studying vitamin D overwhelmingly concluded that low blood serum levels of vitamin D were associated with an increase in overall mortality.

According to the study's authors (Bjelakovic et al. 2014):

'Worst-best case' and 'best-worst case' scenario analyses demonstrated that vitamin D could be associated with a dramatic increase or decrease in mortality.

There are very few natural food sources that provide vitamin D. However, some types of fatty fish, such as mackerel, salmon and tuna can provide a modest amount of vitamin D in the diet—although care must be taken not to intake heavy metals through these fish sources. Small amounts of vitamin D can also be consumed by eating egg yolks, some cheese and liver. The body's primary source for vitamin D comes through exposure to the sun. Unfortunately, recent trends on sun avoidance and the widespread use of sunscreens has contributed to the decline in vitamin D levels among many people.

Testing for vitamin D levels can be critical for determining if you are suffering from a deficiency. However, it is important to understand the different tests available and what they are measuring in your body. There are two measurable forms of vitamin D, including hydroxyvitamin D 25 or "25 (OH) Vitamin D3" which is an inactive form and the "1,25 (OH)" form of which is biologically active. Most doctor-ordered tests only measure the "25 (OH)" form of vitamin D without accounting for the "1,25 (OH)" form that is actually the one that is utilized by your body. Therefore, it is important that you measure both forms when you get tested in order to determine 1) if you are truly deficient in vitamin D or if you are just low in the inactive form of vitamin D and 2) whether or not you are efficiently converting the inactive vitamin D to its biologically active form. It is the job of the kidneys to convert 25(OH) to 1,25(OH) vitamin D, so this can be especially problematic for people with kidney disease of any kind.

*Vitamin E*

Vitamin E naturally occurs in eight different chemical forms, with various levels of biological activity. The alpha form (α-tocopherol) is the most important for human health. In fact, the liver takes up the various forms of vitamin E from the small intestine and preferentially releases the alpha form to the rest of the body (World Health Organization 2014). The primary function of vitamin E in the body is to serve as an antioxidant. Because vitamin E is fat-soluble, it prevents the damage that can occur to the body when it is exposed to oxidized fat. It has also been shown to play an important role in the immune system, proper gene expression and metabolism. The best natural sources of vitamin E include: nuts, seeds, and green leafy vegetables.

*Folate*

Folate is an important water-soluble B vitamin that is critical for synthesizing DNA and RNA as well as in the metabolism of amino acids. Folate is found in a while variety of foods, including green, leafy vegetables, fruit, nuts, legumes, dairy products, meat, eggs and grains. A folate deficiency is most worrisome in women of childbearing age because it may contribute to the risk of giving birth to an infant with a neural tube defect.

*Vitamin K*

Vitamin K is found in two distinct forms, *creatively* called vitamin K1 and vitamin K2. Known for its role in protein clotting and for wreaking havoc in patients who are on prescription blood thinning drugs such as warfarin (Coumadin), research has also shown an important role for vitamin K in maintaining proper bone health and vitamin K deficiencies have been linked to osteoporosis. Vitamin K1 can be found in abundance in green leafy vegetables, avocadoes, tuna, blueberries and blackberries; whereas vitamin K2 is primarily a byproduct of bacterial metabolism and is therefore found in high quantities in many fermented foods and some animal products.

The study of vitamin K has taken a fascinating twist in the last century primarily due to the work of Dr. Weston A. Price. Dr. Price was a dentist who travelled the world examining the diet of indigenous people who experienced superior health and ultimately discovered the importance of a compound he called "Activator X" that is now known to be vitamin K2. It wasn't until 1978 that researchers acknowledged that vitamin K played a role in functions other than blood clotting; that it was in fact a critical component in the course of skeletal metabolism. Today, it is understood that vitamin K1 and K2 play very different roles in the body; K1 is primarily used as a blood clotting protein by the liver, and K2 is important for regulating the deposition of calcium (Masterjohn 2008). In addition, vitamin K2 helps to regulate the activity of both vitamins A and D and is crucial to the proper activity of these key vitamins.

# Understanding Electromagnetic Radiation (EMR)

Electromagnetic radiation is basically an all-encompassing term that is used to describe the energy that is released into space. It is best known as the energy that comes from the stars and the sun, but it is also recognized that common household appliances and electronics are also significant sources for exposure to EMR, including (Zhu et al. 2013):

- Radio waves
- Television sets
- Radar
- Infrared heat
- Regular old lights
- Ultraviolet light (causes sunburns)
- X-rays
- Microwaves (yes, as in a microwave oven)
- Gamma rays

It may help to envision electromagnetic radiation as energy that travels in waves at differing frequencies. Although waves at the beach are not electromagnetic radiation, they illustrate the idea, but at a much slower rate than electromagnetic radiation. For example, waves at the beach may occur at a very low frequency (less than one per second), whereas radio waves can occur at a frequency anywhere from 10,000 to 100,000,000 vibrations per second! While sound is a form of energy that travels in waves, it is not considered electromagnetic radiation because it requires a "medium" to travel through such as air or water, whereas electromagnetic radiation can travel in space.

So, the question becomes "why should we be concerned about our exposure to electromagnetic radiation?"

There is a growing body of evidence demonstrating that the "electrosmog" that is so prevalent in our highly technological society is causing severe health effects. In 2007, teachers at a newly constructed school were found to have a 64 percent increase in the risk of cancer that was ultimately associated with extremely high levels of a particular type of EMF known as "dirty electricity" (Segell 2010). To take it one step further, consider that a property of heavy metals is their great ability to conduct electricity. Therefore, if you have extremely high levels of heavy metals accumulated in the various organs of your body, you may be at an additional risk for adverse health effects due to EMR exposure.

So what you can do to protect yourself from EMR? This is a difficult question because EMR permeates the entire world and is therefore very difficult to avoid. However, small things like minimizing your cell phone use and exposure to WiFi within your home could have long-lasting benefits. Also, removing appliances that generate EMR, such as your microwave, will help to reduce your exposure. Finally, get involved. Contact your local government representatives and let them know you are concerned and that more research needs to be done to help with regulation of EMR.

## Understanding Microbial Biofilms

New research has been shedding light on important "defense mechanisms" that are used by many bacteria and viruses that serve as protective barriers against your own natural defenses as well as medications taken to overcome the infection. Many bacteria, virus and even fungal infections will form what is called "microbial biofilms" around themselves that provides a barrier between them and your immune system, antibiotics and even natural supplements. What's more, these microbial invaders can change and adapt to get better at fighting off your attempts at removing them from your system.

So, how does exposure to heavy metals influence microbial biofilms? It is known that microbes have many of the same requirements for essential minerals as you do, primarily zinc. This means that microbes can become vulnerable when the supply of essential minerals is running low. We already know that many of the heavy metals you are commonly exposed to can cause deficiencies and imbalances in many of the essential minerals—including zinc. You would think this is a good thing! However, microbes have an advantage over us in that they can develop resistance to many toxic heavy metals (de Vicente et al. 1990, Kovac Virsek, Hubad, and Lapanje 2013). This "metal-resistant talent" is due to unique genes within the microbe's DNA that allows them to chemically alter the heavy metals to a form that is less toxic to them and then kick the metals out of their systems (Wagner–Dobler et al. 2000). This trait has proven useful in environmental remediation projects, but in your body it causes a build-up of toxic heavy metals that may provide a further barrier against your attempts to eliminate the infection. What's more, the sticky nature of microbial biofilms attracts toxic metals that are positively charged, which can then link up with the biofilm and provide additional strength.

The following is a list of strategies for reducing or eliminating microbial biofilms that have developed in your body and, along with heavy metals, are continually making you sick (Janossy 2015):

- Digestive enzymes that disrupt the outer layers of the biofilm and expose the hidden microbes.
- Oxygen (for example, through the use of hyperbaric chambers, oxygen drops, face masks, etc.) can disrupt the biofilm colonies that are generally anaerobic in nature.
- EDTA chelation, which removes the heavy metals from the system and weakens the biofilm's tensile strength.
- Supplement with flavonoids, which can suppress the formation of biofilms.
- Ingest charcoal, which is not absorbed through the gut, but can significantly weaken the microbial biofilms.
- Intermittent fasting is beneficial because it deprives the microbes from a continual energy source.

# Chapter 17 References

World Health Organization. 2014. Antimicrobial Resistance: Global Report on Surveillance.

Environmental Protection Agency. 2014. Chemicals evaluated for carcinogenic potential.

Bailey, C. E., C. Y. Hu, Y. N. You, B. K. Bednarski, M. A. Rodriguez-Bigas, J. M. Skibber, S. B. Cantor, and G. J. Chang. 2014. "Increasing Disparities in the Age-Related Incidences of Colon and Rectal Cancers in the United States, 1975-2010." *JAMA surgery*:1-6. doi: 10.1001/jamasurg.2014.1756.

Bjelakovic, G., L. L. Gluud, D. Nikolova, K. Whitfield, J. Wetterslev, R. G. Simonetti, M. Bjelakovic, and C. Gluud. 2014. "Vitamin D supplementation for prevention of mortality in adults." *The Cochrane database of systematic reviews* 1:CD007470. doi: 10.1002/14651858. CD007470.pub3.

Calafat, A. M., X. Ye, L. Y. Wong, A. M. Bishop, and L. L. Needham. 2010. "Urinary concentrations of four parabens in the U.S. population: NHANES 2005-2006." *Environmental health perspectives* 118 (5):679-85. doi: 10.1289/ehp.0901560.

de Vicente, A., M. Aviles, J. C. Codina, J. J. Borrego, and P. Romero. 1990. "Resistance to antibiotics and heavy metals of Pseudomonas aeruginosa isolated from natural waters." *The Journal of applied bacteriology* 68 (6):625-32.

FDA.gov. 2013. "Overview of food ingredients, additives and colors: International food information council (IFIC) and U.S. food and drug administration." Accessed November 23, 2014. http://www.fda.gov/Food/IngredientsPackagingLabeling/FoodAdditivesIngredients/ucm094211.htm - how.

Goetz, A. K., J. C. Rockett, H. Ren, I. Thillainadarajah, and D. J. Dix. 2009. "Inhibition of rat and human steroidogenesis by triazole antifungals." *Systems biology in reproductive medicine* 55 (5-6):214-26. doi: 10.3109/19396360903234045.

Environmental Working Group. 2014. "EWG's 2014 shopper's guide to pesticides in produce." Accessed November 17, 2014. http://www.ewg.org/foodnews/.

National Institutes of Health. 2014. "Vitamin and mineral supplement fact sheets." Accessed November 19, 2014. http://ods.od.nih.gov/factsheets/list-VitaminsMinerals/.

IARC. 2010. Ingested nitrate and nitrite and cyanobacterial peptide toxins. IARC monographs on the evaluation of carcinogenic risks to humans.

Janossy, T. 2015. "Biofilm in lyme, autism, alzheimer's and dementia." Accessed February 13, 2015. http://oradix.com/pages/Biofilm-in-Lyme%2C-Autism%2C-Alzheimer%27s-and-Dementia.html.

Jeong, S. H., B. Y. Kim, H. G. Kang, H. O. Ku, and J. H. Cho. 2005. "Effects of butylated hydroxyanisole on the development and functions of reproductive system in rats." *Toxicology* 208 (1):49-62. doi: 10.1016/j.tox.2004.11.014.

Kovac Virsek, M., B. Hubad, and A. Lapanje. 2013. "Mercury induced community tolerance in microbial biofilms is related to pollution gradients in a long-term polluted river." *Aquatic toxicology* 144-145:208-17. doi: 10.1016/j.aquatox.2013.09.023.

Kresser, C. 2014. "How rebuilding a healthy gut can give you a healthier life." Accessed November 22, 2014. http://chriskresser.com/gut-health.

Masterjohn, C. 2008. "On the trail of the elusive x-factor: a sixty-two-year-old mystery finally solved." Accessed November 1, 2014. http://www.westonaprice.org/abcs-of-nutrition/fat-soluble-activators/.

Mercola, J. 2014. "Vitamin D resource page." Accessed November 20, 2014. http://www.mercola.com/article/vitamin-d-resources.htm.

Mercola, J. 2013a. "How to find the healthiest fare in meat and produce aisles." Accessed November 17, 2014. http://articles.mercola.com/sites/articles/archive/2013/05/08/ewg-pesticide-guide.aspx.

Mercola, J. 2013b. "Resveratrol in grape skins could help treat cancer and more." Accessed November 21, 2014. http://articles.mercola.com/sites/articles/archive/2013/10/28/resveratrol-cancer-prevention.aspx.

Oishi, S. 2002. "Effects of propyl paraben on the male reproductive system." *Food and chemical toxicology: an international journal published for the British Industrial Biological Research Association* 40 (12):1807-13.

Okubo, T., Y. Yokoyama, K. Kano, and I. Kano. 2001. "ER-dependent estrogenic activity of parabens assessed by proliferation of human breast cancer MCF-7 cells and expression of ERalpha and PR." *Food and chemical toxicology: an international journal published for the British Industrial Biological Research Association* 39 (12):1225-32.

Segell, M. 2010. "Is 'electrosmog' harming our health?" Accessed February 7, 2015.

Smith, K. W., I. Souter, I. Dimitriadis, S. Ehrlich, P. L. Williams, A. M. Calafat, and R. Hauser. 2013. "Urinary paraben concentrations and ovarian aging among women from a fertility center." *Environmental health perspectives* 121 (11-12):1299-305. doi: 10.1289/ehp.1205350.

Smith-Spangler, C., M. L. Brandeau, G. E. Hunter, J. C. Bavinger, M. Pearson, P. J. Eschbach, V. Sundaram, H. Liu, P. Schirmer, C. Stave, I. Olkin, and D. M. Bravata. 2012. "Are organic foods safer or healthier than conventional alternatives?: a systematic review." *Annals of internal medicine* 157 (5):348-66. doi: 10.7326/0003-4819-157-5-201209040-00007.

Wagner-Dobler, I., H. Lunsdorf, T. Lubbehusen, H. F. von Canstein, and Y. Li. 2000. "Structure and species composition of mercury-reducing biofilms." *Applied and environmental microbiology* 66 (10):4559-63.

Zhu, M., G. Nie, H. Meng, T. Xia, A. Nel, and Y. Zhao. 2013. "Physicochemical properties determine nanomaterial cellular uptake, transport, and fate." *Accounts of chemical research* 46 (3):622-31. doi: 10.1021/ar300031y.

# CHAPTER 18

# Preventing Disease with Lifestyle Changes!

Now that you have put in the time and effort necessary to overcome heavy metal poisoning, it is important to understand the many ways you can ensure that your health is not compromised again! It is extremely difficult to completely avoid exposure to toxic heavy metals in the highly polluted environment we live in today. However, there are several steps that can be taken to improve your ability to successfully manage and prevent heavy metal exposures.

The following tools are simple methods that can be incorporated into your daily lifestyle that will provide continual preventive measures against future heavy metal exposure.

*Regularly scheduled testing for heavy metals*

We've mentioned the importance of being tested for heavy metals in order to identify their role in wreaking havoc with your health. So, you may ask why it is also listed in the chapter on prevention? The answer is to maintain your vigilance. Remember that exposure to heavy metals can often times occur without your knowledge. These are silent killers that make their way into your body in stealthy ways. A great way to make sure that you are protected against future health problems that are due to heavy metals is to be regularly tested for them. I recommend that you be tested at least once per year.

*Far infrared saunas*

Your skin is another crucial organ for eliminating the "bad" stuff from your body. A great way to improve the effectiveness of your skin in the detoxification process is to improve your efficiency and frequency of sweating. Far infrared saunas are a great tool that can be used to enhance the detoxification process and as such can also be an important preventive measure against accumulating heavy metals in your system. In addition to assisting with the process of sweating, saunas can improve the metabolic processes as well as improve circulation.

Far infrared saunas differ from more traditional saunas in the type of energy that is used to increase your body temperature. The heat waves of a far infrared sauna penetrate the body directly and are therefore able to heat the tissues more deeply and raise the body core temperature effectively. In contrast, a traditional sauna is a heated environment that warms the body from the outside. Both types of saunas will result in a significant amount of sweating, but the far infrared sauna will do so at a lower temperature. Also, because the infrared sauna is heating your body directly (as opposed to just heating your environment) often times they are more comfortable and the difficulty breathing that is often associated with more traditional saunas can be avoided.

*Eating fermented foods/gut health*

Ok, we have mentioned the importance of maintaining good gut health a number of times. But, it is worth reminding you that the first and foremost pathway for eliminating unwanted items from your body is through defecation! If your gastrointestinal system is not functioning properly, pretty soon neither will any other system. Your gut is the first line of defense. You can improve the elimination capacity of your gastrointestinal tract, liver and kidneys by supplementing with methionine, vitamin B12 and n-acetylcysteine. Finally, you can slow the absorption of heavy metals through the gastrointestinal tract by increasing total dietary fiber intake and remaining sufficiently hydrated (drink 60-90 ounces of clean water daily). Supplementation with bentonite as well as consuming certain foods such as beans, whole grain breads and cereals may also help to minimize the absorption of heavy metals.

*Regular exercise*

Similar to the preventive measures achieved through the use of an infrared sauna, exercise can help prevent heavy metal poisoning by increasing your sweat time. But, the benefits of exercise extend beyond simply sweating more. You will see improvements in your mental clarity and outlook from regular exercise. Maintaining an ideal weight will prove easier, and the effort required to fit an exercise program into your schedule may just provide you with motivation to improve other areas of your life, such as diet and stress levels. It's a win win!

### *Identify And Avoid Exposure As Much As Possible*

Evaluation of your immediate and controllable surroundings will help you to determine the most likely sources of exposure. You may want to consider testing your water, evaluating your cooking utensils and bake ware, evaluating the building materials that have been used in your home, eating only organic fruits and vegetables, eating fish with caution and ensuring your supplements come from highly reputable sources. In addition, including certain supplements such as vitamin C and lipoic acid can help prevent damage that is caused by exposure to heavy metals due to their powerful antioxidant properties.

### *Consider Continual Oral or Intravenous Chelation Therapy*

Continuing chelation therapy even after the initial crisis due to heavy metals has been dealt with is an important tool for preventing future exposure to heavy metals from

## Gluten Free Food List

- Healthy fats such as extra virgin olive oil, sesame oil and coconut oil
- Protein sources such as whole eggs, grass-fed meat, fowl, poultry, and wild game.
- Vegetables
- Low-sugar Fruit: avocado, bell peppers, cucumber, tomato, zucchini, squash, pumpkin, eggplant, lemons, limes.
- Herbs, seasonings, and condiments
- Non-gluten grains such as amaranth, buckwheat, rice, millet, quinoa, sorghum, certified gluten-free oats
- Legumes (beans, lentils, peas)
- Whole sweet fruit: berries are best
- Cow's milk and cream
- Cottage cheese, yogurt, and kefir
- Sweeteners: natural stevia
- Wine

accumulating in your body. In many cases, your natural detoxification system is overwhelmed or simply cannot remove the heavy metals fast enough to prevent damage from occurring. Chelation therapy is a safe way to eliminate heavy metals from your system quickly and efficiently.

### Go Gluten Free!

You may be wondering how adoption of a gluten-free diet will help prevent heavy metal toxicity. There are many very valid reasons for removing gluten from your diet, but from the perspective of preventing heavy metal toxicity you have to consider its impact on the detox organs and the immune system in particular. You don't have to be one of the 1 percent of individuals who have clinically been diagnosed as having celiac disease—an autoimmune disorder—to suffer adverse health effects from the consumption of gluten.

You may recall from our discussion about our natural detoxification pathways the extreme importance of your liver. There is mounting evidence that consumption of gluten can contribute to liver damage. There are two primary reasons that gluten causes damage to the liver: 1) increased permeability in the intestinal lining. This results in the absorption of compounds (perhaps heavy metals) into the blood stream that would normally be filtered out by an intact gastrointestinal system. The body's response to foreign compounds in the blood stream is to launch an immune system attack! The immune system assault is nonselective and in general does not take prisoners. Damage to the liver can be a serious side effect, including elevated liver enzymes, inflammation and scarring, and 2) when gluten irritates the gut lining, it is not just environmental toxicants that can inadvertently cross into the blood, but food and bacteria toxins that would normally be eliminated through the bowels. This places added stress on the liver as it attempts to detoxify this increased assault on the body. When the liver is taxed, you are more susceptible to the adverse effects of heavy metal exposure.

"...eating too much gluten, whether you're gluten sensitive or not, tends to have an effect on the intestines. It can create a condition in the intestine known as intestinal permeability, or what in common lay terms is referred to as leaky gut."

-Dr. Peter Osborne (The "Gluten Warrior," Author and Academic)

# CHAPTER 19

# Heavy Metals and Your Pets

## Heavy Metals and Pets

Heavy metals are not just toxic for humans. Animals suffer from adverse health effects in many of the same ways—and from many of the same sources! In fact, a recent survey of dog and cat treats showed shockingly high levels of lead, mercury and cadmium (Adams 2014). The FDA has also warned about contaminated pet food:

> Since 2007, FDA has become aware of an increasing number of illnesses in pets associated with the consumption of jerky pet treats. As of September 24, 2013, FDA has received approximately 3000 reports of pet illnesses, which may be related to consumption of the jerky treats. The reports involve more than 3600 dogs, 10 cats and include more than 580 deaths.

While the FDA recognizes the risk of contaminated food for pets, it has not established any limits for heavy metals; therefore, pet food manufacturers can legally sale products regardless of the presence of heavy metals. This is true even for certified organic pet food, which is unregulated by the USDA (Adams 2014). Equally troublesome is the huge cost associated with treating a pet for heavy metal toxicity. A study conducted by the VPI pet insurance company in California estimated that poisoning caused by heavy metals resulted claims averaging $952 dollars (DVM360 Magazine 2010)! An additional study comparing the various forms of dog and cat food for heavy metal content came to the following conclusions (Atkins 2011):

- There is a trend toward higher metal content in dry versus wet pet food, especially for strontium, aluminum and lead
- Price, perceived quality and overall ratings did not predict the presence or absence of heavy metals
- There was no evidence that foods containing higher amounts of fish also had higher levels of heavy metals

Heavy metal toxicity in a dog or cat will cause symptoms that range from convulsions, hyperactivity, and GI issues, to awkward movements and weakness. In addition, exposure to heavy metals such as mercury can increase the risk for seizures in animals. Rodents kept as pets can be especially vulnerable to the effects of heavy metal exposure. Lead can present a particular problem if the pet is kept completely indoors and the living quarters have been painted with lead-based paint. Symptoms of lead poisoning in rodents may include unusual body positioning due to abdominal pain, nervousness, vomiting, diarrhea, and stumbling (Petco 2014).

Birds can also be susceptible to heavy metal poisoning, particularly iron, lead and zinc. Exposure may lead to symptoms of depression, incoordination, constant thirst, and tremors (Becker 2010).

## Chapter 19 References

Adams, M. 2014. "Pet treats found contaminated with heavy metals--Health Ranger releases shocking data on lead, mercury and cadmium in dog and cat treats." Accessed November 21, 2014. http://www.naturalnews.com/044795_pet_treats_toxic_heavy_metals_made_in_china.html.

Atkins, P. 2011. Analysis of pet food for inorganic contaminants. SPEXCertiPrep.

Becker, K. 2010. "Common ways your pet can be poisoned." Accessed November 21, 2014. http://healthypets.mercola.com/sites/healthypets/archive/2010/09/07/common-pet-poisons-present-in-households.aspx.

DVM360 Magazine. 2010. VPI pet insurance counts the poisons that send dogs to the veterinary hospital. Accessed November 21, 2014. http://veterinarynews.dvm360.com/blue-buffalo-issues-voluntary-pet-food-recall?rel=canonical

Petco. 2014. "Hamster care--heavy metals." Accessed November 21, 2014. http://www.petco.com/Content/ArticleList/Article/33/20/861/Heavy-Metals.aspx.

# Appendices

## FAQ's
## What are heavy metals?

In general, the term "heavy metals" refers to a group of metals and metalloid compounds that share similar characteristics and have the capacity to cause adverse health effects. Heavy metals occur in the environment both from natural and anthropogenic practices and have become a widespread concern. While some heavy metals are essential for normal physiology at specific concentrations, many heavy metals have no known benefit to human health.

## Should I be tested for heavy metal poisoning?

Yes. Because heavy metals have become a widespread problem in the environment, exposure is a common occurrence. Also, many heavy metals accumulate in the body, which means that even low exposures can lead to significant health problems over time. The only way to know your particular body burden of heavy metals is to be tested. I recommend that everyone be tested at least once per year if results are normal. However, if your test results come back showing that you have issues with one or more heavy metal then more frequent testing may be necessary until the issue is resolved through treatment.

## What is chelation therapy?

Chelation therapy is the utilization of chelating agents, which tightly bind to metals and allows them to be eliminated from the body. In the world of allopathic medicine, chelation therapy is primarily used to treat acute cases of heavy metal poisoning. It is also gaining recognition among practitioners of integrative medicine for the treatment of long-term heavy metal exposure as well as in the prevention of certain chronic diseases such as cardiovascular disease.

*Dr. Pamela J Owens*

## How can I prevent heavy metal exposure?

Knowledge is key to minimizing the risk of exposure. Understanding where heavy metals are typically "hidden" and eliminating those items from your surroundings and food supply is important to prevent unwanted exposures. Organizations such as the Environmental Working Group provide information that is regularly updated on the safety of common household items regarding issues such as the presence of heavy metals. Also, regular testing for heavy metals is a great way of ensuring that any inadvertent exposures can be dealt with early—before adverse health effects are observed.

# Abstracts from Cutting Edge Research in Heavy Metals Toxicology

*Mercury In Breast Milk - A Health Hazard For Infants In Gold Mining Areas?*

Int J Hyg Environ Health. 2008 Oct; 211(5-6):615-23. doi: 10.1016/j. ijheh.2007.09.015.
Bose-O'Reilly S, Lettmeier B, Roider G, Siebert U, Drasch G.

## Abstract

Breast-feeding can be a source of mercury exposure for infants. The main concern up to now is methyl-mercury exposure of women at child-bearing age. Certain fish species have high levels of methyl-mercury leading to consumer's advisory guidelines in regard of fish consumption to protect infants from mercury exposure passing through breast milk. Little is known about the transfer of inorganic mercury passing through breast milk to infants. Epidemiological studies showed negative health effects of inorganic mercury in gold mining areas. Small-scale gold miners use mercury to extract the gold from the ore. Environmental and health assessments of gold mining areas in Indonesia, Tanzania and Zimbabwe showed a high exposure with inorganic mercury in these gold mining areas, and a negative health impact of the exposure to the miners and the communities. This paper reports about the analysis and the results of 46 breast milk samples collected from mercury-exposed mothers. The median level of 1.87mug/l is fairly high compared to other results from literature. Some breast milk samples showed very high levels of mercury (up to 149mug/l). Fourteen of the 46 breast milk samples exceed 4mug/l which is considered to be a "high" level. US EPA recommends a "Reference Dose" of 0.3mug inorganic mercury/kg body weight/day [United States Environmental Protection Agency, 1997. Volume V: Health Effects of Mercury and Mercury Compounds. Study Report EPA-452/R-97-007: US EPA]. Twenty-two of the 46 children from these gold mining areas had a higher calculated total mercury uptake. The highest calculated daily mercury uptake of 127mg exceeds by far the recommended maximum uptake of inorganic mercury. Further systematic research of mercury in breast milk from small-scale gold mining areas is needed to increase the knowledge about the bio-transfer of mercury from mercury vapor-exposed mothers passing through breast milk to the breast-fed infant.

*Association Of Oxidative Stress With Arsenic Methylation In Chronic Arsenic-Exposed Children And Adults*

Toxicol Appl Pharmacol. 2008 Oct 1;232(1):142-9. doi: 10.1016/j. taap.2008.06.010. Epub 2008 Jul 1.
Xu Y[1], Wang Y, Zheng Q, Li X, Li B, Jin Y, Sun X, Sun G.

## Abstract

Though oxidative stress is recognized as an important pathogenic mechanism of arsenic, and arsenic methylation capacity is suggested to be highly involved in arsenic-related diseases, the association of arsenic methylation capacity with arsenic-induced oxidative stress remains unclear. To explore oxidative stress and its association with arsenic methylation, cross-sectional studies were conducted among 208 high and 59 low arsenic-exposed subjects. Levels of urinary arsenic species [inorganic arsenic (iAs), monomethylated arsenic (MMA) and dimethylated arsenic (DMA)] were determined by hydride generation atomic absorption spectrometry. Proportions of urinary arsenic species, the first methylation ratio (FMR) and the secondary methylation ratio (SMR) were used as indicators for arsenic methylation capacity. Urinary 8-hydroxy-2'-deoxyguanosine (8-OHdG) concentrations were analyzed by enzyme-linked immunosorbent assay kits. Reduced glutathione (GSH) levels and superoxide dismutase (SOD) activity in whole blood were determined to reflect anti-oxidative status. The high arsenic-exposed children and adults were significantly increased in urinary 8-OHdG concentrations but decreased in blood GSH levels compared with the low exposed children and adults. In multiple linear regression models, blood GSH levels and urinary 8-OHdG concentrations of arsenic-exposed children and adults showed strong associations with the levels of urinary arsenic species. Arsenic-exposed subjects in the lower and the upper quartiles of proportions of urinary arsenic species, FMR or SMR were significantly different in urinary 8-OHdG, blood GSH and SOD. The associations of arsenic methylation capacity with 8-OHdG, GSH and SOD were also observed in multivariate regression analyses. These results may provide linkage between arsenic methylation capacity and oxidative stress in humans and suggest that adverse health effects induced by arsenic are related to arsenic methylation through oxidative stress.

*Dr. Pamela J Owens*

*Toxic Metal And Nicotine Content Of Cigarettes Sold In China, 2009 And 2012*

Tob Control. 2014 Oct 21. pii: tobaccocontrol-2014-051804. doi: 10.1136/tobaccocontrol-2014-051804. [Epub ahead of print]
O'Connor RJ, Schneller LM, Caruso RV, Stephens WE, Li Q, Yuan J, Fong GT.

## Abstract

## BACKGROUND:

Metals of primary health concern can accumulate in the tobacco plant and contribute to smokers' exposures to carcinogens, a significant cause of the millions of smoking-related deaths in China each year. These exposures are due to the smoker's addiction to nicotine.

## OBJECTIVE:

This study sought to explore toxic heavy metal and nicotine concentrations in the tobacco of Chinese cigarette brands purchased in 2009 and 2012, as well as its regional variation.

## METHODS:

Cigarette packs for this study were purchased from seven Chinese cities in 2009 and 2012, and 91 pairs of cigarettes were matched based on UPC for comparison. Ten cigarette sticks were randomly selected from each pack and tested using polarised energy dispersive X-ray fluorescence (XRF) for arsenic (As), cadmium (Cd), chromium (Cr), nickel (Ni) and lead (Pb) concentrations. Nicotine analysis was conducted following Coresta's Recommended Method N°62. Data analysis was conducted using SPSS, encompassing descriptive statistics, correlations and generalised estimating equations to observe changes in brand varieties overtime.

## FINDINGS:

On average, from 2009 to 2012, As, Cd, Cr and Pb concentrations have decreased in Chinese tobacco. Of the seven cities where the cigarette brands were purchased, only four cities showed significant differences of the selected metals from 2009 to 2012. However, there was no significant change in the tobacco nicotine content from 2009 to 2012.

## CONCLUSIONS:

Tobacco in Chinese cigarettes purchased in seven geographically disbursed cities contains consistently high levels of metals, including carcinogens like Cd. One source may be the improper use of fertilizers. These numbers should be monitored more carefully and regulated by health officials.

*Dr. Pamela J Owens*

*Effect Of A Single Dose Of Cadmium On Pregnant Wistar Rats And Their Offspring*

Reprod Domest Anim. 2014 Oct 17. doi: 10.1111/rda.12439. [Epub ahead of print]
Díaz MD[1], González N, Gómez S, Quiroga M, Najle R, Barbeito C.

## Abstract

Cadmium (Cd) is a well-known toxicant targeting many organs, among them placenta. This heavy metal also has embryonary and foetal toxicity. This study was undertaken to analyse the effect of a single Cd dose administered at 4, 7, 10 or 15 days of gestation on the offspring of pregnant rats sacrificed at 20 days of gestation. Cadmium chloride was administered subcutaneously at 10 mg/kg body weight to Wistar pregnant dams; control animals received a proportionate volume of sterile normal saline by the same route. Maternal uteri, livers, kidneys and lungs, and foetuses were examined at necropsy. Samples of maternal organs and whole foetuses were collected for histopathologic examination, determination of Cd levels and staining by the Alizarin red S technique. Results revealed a clear embryotoxic and a teratogenic effect of this heavy metal, the former as a significant increase in the number of resorptions, and the latter as significant decrease of the gestational sac weight, and the size and weight of foetuses of Cd-treated dams as well as induced malformations in skull bones, vertebrae and thoracic, and pelvian limbs. The deleterious effects found were similar to those previously reported for other animal models suggesting a high conservation of the pathogenic mechanisms of Cd. Additionally, many of the addressed aspects showed a slight dependence on the time of administration of the toxic that might be due to the accumulation of the metal in different organs, as we were able to demonstrate by the analysis of its concentration.

*Effects Of Environmental Temperature Change On Mercury Absorption In Aquatic Organisms With Respect To Climate Warming*

J Toxicol Environ Health A. 2014;77(22-24):1477-90. doi:10.1080/15287394.2014.955892.
Pack EC[1], Lee SH, Kim CH, Lim CH, Sung DG, Kim MH, Park KH, Lim KM, Choi DW, Kim SW.

## Abstract

Because of global warming, the quantity of naturally generated mercury (Hg) will increase, subsequently methylation of Hg existing in seawater may be enhanced, and the content of metal in marine products rise which consequently results in harm to human health. Studies of the effects of temperatures on Hg absorption have not been adequate. In this study, in order to observe the effects of temperature changes on Hg absorption, inorganic Hg or methylmercury (MeHg) was added to water tanks containing loaches. Loach survival rates decreased with rising temperatures, duration, and exposure concentrations in individuals exposed to inorganic Hg and MeHg. The MeHg-treated group died sooner than the inorganic Hg-exposed group. The total Hg and MeHg content significantly increased with temperature and time in both metal-exposed groups. The MeHg-treated group had higher metal absorption rates than inorganic Hg-treated loaches. The correlation coefficients for temperature elevation and absorption were significant in both groups. The results of this study may be used as basic data for assessing in vivo hazards from environmental changes such as climate warming.

*Dr. Pamela J Owens*

*Clinically Approved Iron Chelators Influence Zebrafish Mortality, Hatching Morphology And Cardiac Function*

PLoS One. 2014 Oct 16;9(10):e109880. doi: 10.1371/journal.pone.0109880. eCollection 2014.
Hamilton JL[1], Hatef A[2], Imran Ul-Haq M[1], Nair N[2], Unniappan S[2], Kizhakkedathu JN[3].

## Abstract

Iron chelation therapy using iron (III) specific chelators such as desferrioxamine (DFO, Desferal), deferasirox (Exjade or ICL-670), and deferiprone (Ferriprox or L1) are the current standard of care for the treatment of iron overload. Although each chelator is capable of promoting some degree of iron excretion, these chelators are also associated with a wide range of well documented toxicities. However, there is currently very limited data available on their effects in developing embryos. In this study, we took advantage of the rapid development and transparency of the zebrafish embryo, Danio rerio to assess and compare the toxicity of iron chelators. All three iron chelators described above were delivered to zebrafish embryos by direct soaking and their effects on mortality, hatching and developmental morphology were monitored for 96 hpf. To determine whether toxicity was specific to embryos, we examined the effects of chelator exposure via intra peritoneal injection on the cardiac function and gene expression in adult zebrafish. Chelators varied significantly in their effects on embryo mortality, hatching and morphology. While none of the embryos or adults exposed to DFO were negatively affected, ICL -treated embryos and adults differed significantly from controls, and L1 exerted toxic effects in embryos alone. ICL-670 significantly increased the mortality of embryos treated with doses of 0.25 mM or higher and also affected embryo morphology, causing curvature of larvae treated with concentrations above 0.5 mM. ICL-670 exposure (10 μL of 0.1 mM injection) also significantly increased the heart rate and cardiac output of adult zebrafish. While L1 exposure did not cause toxicity in adults, it did cause morphological defects in embryos at 0.5 mM. This study provides first evidence on iron chelator toxicity in early development and will help to guide our approach on better understanding the mechanism of iron chelator toxicity.

*Gastrointestinal Absorption Of Uranium Compounds - A Review*

Regul Toxicol Pharmacol. 2014 Sep 28. pii: S0273-2300(14)00192-5. doi: 10.1016/j.yrtph.2014.08.012. [Epub ahead of print]
Konietzka R.

## Abstract

Uranium occurs naturally in soil and rocks, and therefore where it is present in water-soluble form it also occurs naturally in groundwater as well as in drinking water obtained from groundwater. Animal studies suggest that the toxicity of uranium is mainly due to its damage to kidney tubular cells following exposure to soluble uranium compounds. The assessments of the absorption of uranium via the gastrointestinal tract vary, and this has consequences for regulation, in particular the derivation of e.g. drinking water limit values. Absorption rates vary according to the nature and solubility of the compound in which uranium is presented to the test animals and depending on the animal species used in the test. No differences for sex have been observed for absorption in either animals or humans. However, human biomonitoring data do show that boys excrete significantly more uranium than girls. In animal studies neonates took up more uranium than adults or older children. Nutritional status, and in particular the iron content of the diet, have a marked influence on absorption, and higher uranium levels in food intake also appear to increase the absorption rate. If the pointers to an absorption mechanism competing with iron are correct, these mechanisms could also explain the relatively high concentration and chemical toxicity of uranium in the kidneys. It is here (and in the duodenum) that divalent metal transporter 1 (DMT1), which is primarily responsible for the passage of iron (or uranium?) through the cell membranes, is most strongly expressed.

*Dr. Pamela J Owens*

*Evaluation Of Toxic Metals And Essential Elements In Children With Learning Disabilities From A Rural Area Of Southern Brazil*

Int J Environ Res Public Health. 2014 Oct 17;11(10):10806-23. doi: 10.3390/ijerph111010806.
Nascimento SN, Charão MF, Moro AM, Roehrs M, Paniz C, Baierle M, Brucker N, Gioda A, Jr FB, Bohrer D, Avila DS, Garcia SC.

## Abstract

Children's exposure to metals can result in adverse effects such as cognitive function impairments. This study aimed to evaluate some toxic metals and levels of essential trace elements in blood, hair, and drinking water in children from a rural area of Southern Brazil. Cognitive ability and δ-aminolevulinate dehydratase (ALA-D) activity were evaluated. Oxidative stress was evaluated as a main mechanism of metal toxicity, through the quantification of malondialdehyde (MDA) levels. This study included 20 children from a rural area and 20 children from an urban area. Our findings demonstrated increase in blood lead (Pb) levels (BLLs). Also, increased levels of nickel (Ni) in blood and increase of aluminum (Al) levels in hair and drinking water in rural children were found. Deficiency in selenium (Se) levels was observed in rural children as well. Rural children with visual-motor immaturity presented Pb levels in hair significantly increased in relation to rural children without visual-motor immaturity ($p < 0.05$). Negative correlations between BLLs and ALA-D activity and positive correlations between BLLs and ALA-RE activity were observed. MDA was significantly higher in rural compared to urban children ($p < 0.05$). Our findings suggest that rural children were co-exposed to toxic metals, especially Al, Pb and Ni. Moreover, a slight deficiency of Se was observed. Low performance on cognitive ability tests and ALA-D inhibition can be related to metal exposure in rural children. Oxidative stress was suggested as a main toxicological mechanism involved in metal exposure.

*Biomedical Implications Of Heavy Metals Induced Imbalances In Redox Systems*

Biomed Res Int. 2014;2014:640754. doi: 10.1155/2014/640754. Epub 2014 Aug 12.
Sharma B[1], Singh S[2], Siddiqi NJ[3].

## Abstract

Several workers have extensively worked out the metal induced toxicity and have reported the toxic and carcinogenic effects of metals in human and animals. It is well known that these metals play a crucial role in facilitating normal biological functions of cells as well. One of the major mechanisms associated with heavy metal toxicity has been attributed to generation of reactive oxygen and nitrogen species, which develops imbalance between the prooxidant elements and the antioxidants (reducing elements) in the body. In this process, a shift to the former is termed as oxidative stress. The oxidative stress mediated toxicity of heavy metals involves damage primarily to liver (hepatotoxicity), central nervous system (neurotoxicity), DNA (genotoxicity), and kidney (nephrotoxicity) in animals and humans. Heavy metals are reported to impact signaling cascade and associated factors leading to apoptosis. The present review illustrates an account of the current knowledge about the effects of heavy metals (mainly arsenic, lead, mercury, and cadmium) induced oxidative stress as well as the possible remedies of metal(s) toxicity through natural/ synthetic antioxidants, which may render their effects by reducing the concentration of toxic metal(s). This paper primarily concerns the clinicopathological and biomedical implications of heavy metals induced oxidative stress and their toxicity management in mammals.

*Dr. Pamela J Owens*

*EDTA Chelation Therapy, Without Added Vitamin C, Decreases Oxidative DNA Damage And Lipid Peroxidation*

Altern Med Rev. 2009 Mar;14(1):56-61.
Roussel AM, Hininger-Favier I, Waters RS, Osman M, Fernholz K, Anderson RA.

## Abstract

Chelation therapy is thought to not only remove contaminating metals but also to decrease free radical production. However, in standard ethylene diamine tetracetic acid (EDTA) chelation therapy, high doses of vitamin C with potential pro-oxidant effects are often added to the chelation solution. The authors demonstrated previously that the intravenous administration of the standard chelation cocktail, containing high amounts of vitamin C, resulted in an acute transitory pro-oxidant burst that should be avoided in the treatment of pathologies at risk of increased oxidative stress such as diabetes and cardiovascular disease. The current study was designed to determine the acute and chronic biochemical effects of chelation therapy on accepted clinical, antioxidant variables. An EDTA chelation cocktail not containing ascorbic acid was administered to six adult patients for five weeks (10 sessions of chelation therapy); antioxidant indicators were monitored. Immediately after the initial chelation session, in contrast with the data previously reported with the standard cocktail containing high doses of vitamin C, none of the oxidative stress markers were adversely modified. After five weeks, plasma peroxide levels, monitored by malondialdehyde, decreased by 20 percent, and DNA damage, monitored by formamidopyrimidine-DNA glycosylase (Fpg) sensitive sites, decreased by 22 percent. Remaining antioxidant-related variables did not change. In summary, this study demonstrates that multiple sessions of EDTA chelation therapy in combination with vitamins and minerals, but without added ascorbic acid, decreases oxidative stress. These results should be beneficial in the treatment of diseases associated with increased oxidative stress such as diabetes and cardiovascular diseases.

# Glossary

**Adjuvants:** An agent that is used to modify the effects of other agents, typically for pharmacological or immunological uses.

**Amalgam:** A mixture of mercury and other metals; typically used to fill cavities in teeth.

**Anti-nutrient:** A compound that interferes with the absorption of vitamins, minerals or other nutrients.

**Atherosclerosis:** An occlusion of the arteries that may result in myocardial infarction (heart attack) or stroke.

**Autoimmunity:** A pathological condition in which the immune system mistakes an organism's native molecules as being foreign and mounts an immune response.

**Blood brain barrier:** A barrier between the circulating blood and the brain that is designed to protect the brain from contaminants that may be present in the blood.

**Celiac Disease:** An autoimmune disease that is caused by an immune response that is initiated following the ingestion of gluten.

**Detoxification:** The process by which the body converts toxicant from a toxic state to a safe form that can be eliminated from the body.

**Epigenetics:** Modifications to DNA that turn genes "on" or "off." Evidence is increasingly showing that epigenetics can be passed down from one generation to the next.

**Free radicals:** An atom, molecule or ion with an unpaired electron. Free radicals are extremely reactive and can cause extensive damage within biological systems.

**Gluten Intolerance:** A spectrum of disorders in which gluten has adverse effects on the body.

**Half-life:** the amount of time required for a quantity to fall to half its value as measured at the beginning of the time period.

**Hypertension:** A clinical term for high blood pressure.

**Methylmercury:** The organic form of mercury that most easily accumulates in biological systems.

**Neuropathy:** Damage or a disease that affects the nerves.

**Neurotoxin:** A substance that inhibits the proper functions of neurons.

**Omega-3 Fatty Acids:** An essential fatty acid that cannot be synthesized by the body, also called linolenic acids.

**Oxidative Stress:** A stressful situation that occurs when the body's production of free radicals overwhelms the body's system to overcome or eliminate them.

**Permeability:** The ability of a membrane to transmit fluids from one side to another.

**Sub-lethal:** Not sufficient to cause death.

**Vertigo:** A sensation of spinning that is related to problems of the inner ear.

# Dr. Owens Recommended Websites for Further Information and Products

Dr. Pamela Owens www.drpamowens.com/blog &
    www.drpamelaowens.com
    Email: drpjowens@atmc.net and drpjowens@gmail.com
Dr. Karen Becker www.healthypets.mercola.com &
    www.drkarenbecker.com
Suzy Cohen, RPh www.SuzyCohen.com &
    www.ScriptEssentials.com
Dr. Carolyn Dean www.drcarolyndean.com
Dr. Garry Gordon www.gordonresearch.com &
    www.longevityplus.com
Dr. Ron Grisanti www.functionalmedicineuniversity.com &
    www.yourmedicaldetective.com
Dr. Roy Heilbron Holistic Cardiology See my you tube at
    https://www.youtube.com/watch?v=6UyDmDdfEjU
    Email: Heilbron@mac.com
Dr. Marty Hinz www.neurosciencemyths.com
Dr. Richard Horowitz http://www.richardihorowitz.md.com
Dr. Mark Hyman www.drhyman.com
Dr. Thomas Janossy www.oradix.com
Dr. Daniel Kalish www.kalishinstitute.com & www.kalishwellness
Dr. Datis Kharrazian www.brainhealthbook.com &
    www.thyroidbook.com
Dr. Ben Lynch www.mthfr.net
Dr. Sue Massie
    www.naturesgardenofhealth.com
    Email: suemassie45@aol.com
Dr. Joe Mercola www.mercola.com
Dr. Peter Osborne www.towncenterwellness.com &
    www.glutenfreesociety.org
Dr. John Palmer www.palmerdmd.com
Dr. David Perlmutter www.drperlmutter.com & www.perlhealth.com
Dr. Sonia Rapaport www.havenmedical.com
Dr. Sherry Rogers www.prestigepublishing.com
Dr. Chris Shade www.quicksilverscientific.com

Dr. Ritchie Shoemaker www.survivingmold.com
Suzanne Somers www.suzannesomers.com
Dr. Neal Speight www.centerforwellness.com
J.J.Virgin, CNS, CHFS www.jjvirgin.com

# About the Author

Pamela Owens, DC, FIAMA, ND and CFMP, is not only a successful Chiropractic Physician, but also one of America's Foremost Toxic Metal Experts. She tests hundreds of people every year for toxic heavy metals and has been very successful in helping improve their quality of life. She also has extensive training in Naturopathic Medicine & Acupuncture, utilizing nutrition, vitamin supplements, environmental toxicity testing, and awareness--as well as personal consultations. She encourages lifestyle changes to promote healthy living and as Anthony Robbins would say: she "walks the talk." Dr. Owens is well respected in her community and often voted the best alternative physician. She was recently featured on CBS, NBC, FOX, and ABC news for her achievements.

Dr. Owens graduated from Logan Chiropractic College in 1989 and went into private practice in St. Louis, MO. After many years, she returned home to North Carolina and continues to practice. Her expertise has expanded to include board certification in Acupuncture through the International Academy of Medical Acupuncture. She has received numerous post graduate certifications including: Certified Functional Medicine Practitioner, The Kalish Method, Manipulation under Anesthesia, Spinal Rehabilitation and Laser & Electrical Auricular therapy. With Dr. Owens, continuing education is an ongoing part of her drive to help as many people as possible and encourage them to make their life healthier.

*Please visit Dr. Owens' website and blog at: www.drpamelaowens. com www.drpamowens.com/blog and refer your family and friends to share this important information today!!*

*Please like us on Facebook and Google + help spread the word!*

Dr. Pamela J. Owens

# Index

Printed in the United States
By Bookmasters